Editors   Moustapha Hamdi
Dennis C. Hammond
Foad Nahai

Vertical Scar Mammaplasty

Editors Moustapha Hamdi
Dennis C. Hammond
Foad Nahai

Vertical Scar Mammaplasty

With 163 Figures, Mostly in Colour,
and 7 Tables

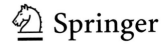 Springer

Editors

Moustapha Hamdi, MD, FCCP
University Hospital of Gent
Department of Plastic Surgery
De Pintelaan 185
9000 Gent, Belgium

Dennis C. Hammond, MD
Center for Breast and Body Contouring
4070 Lake Drive
Grand Rapids, MI 49546, USA

Foad Nahai, MD
Paces Plastic Surgery & Recovery Center
3200 Downwood Circle
Atlanta, GA 30327, USA

ISBN 3-540-22101-8
Springer Verlag Berlin Heidelberg New York

Library of Congress Control Number: 2004110371

Springer is a part of Springer Science + Business Media

springeronline.com

© Springer-Verlag Berlin Heidelberg 2005
Printed in Germany

The use of general descriptive names, registered names, trademarks, etc. in this publication does not imply, even in the absence of a specific statement, that such names are exempt from the relevant protective laws and regulations and therefore free for general use.

Product liability: The publishers cannot guarantee the accuracy of any information about dosage and application contained in this book. In every individual case the user must check such information by consulting the relevant literature.

Editor: Gabriele Schröder, Heidelberg
Desk editor: Irmela Bohn, Heidelberg
Production: ProEdit GmbH, Elke Beul-Göhringer, Heidelberg
Cover design: Estudio Calamar, F. Steinen-Broo, Pau/Girona, Spain
Typesetting and reproduction of the figures: AM-productions GmbH, Wiesloch
Printing: ABC-Druck GmbH, Heidelberg
Binding: Litges & Dopf, Heppenheim

Printed on acid-free paper
24/3150beu-göh   5 4 3 2 1 0

Preface 1

Aesthetic improvement and scar reduction has become the new front line in breast reduction surgery. It is probably easier to show surgeons who have spent many years honing their skills how to modify their own techniques to optimize scarring and achieve a better aesthetic outcome than to convince them to learn a new technique.

I have tried in this book to assemble the techniques and thought processes involved in the evolution of the vertical scar mammaplasty over the last 10 years. It is a worthy attempt to draw on the cumulative experience of master surgeons and mentors in order to increase our chances of obtaining the best possible results. Each chapter represents an individual author's personal approach to breast reduction using various pedicles. A treasure trove of previously untapped information is contained within these pages; the invited authors share their personal thoughts, explain how they refine their results, and take the reader through the critical planning process essential to achieving optimal results.

I was lucky enough to be trained in Brussels when it was the preeminent center for practicing the vertical scar mammaplasty. In the early 1990s, I watched the technique evolve, first through the dedication and efforts of Madeleine Lejour and later by her followers at the Free University of Brussels. During this time I was taught to perform the vertical scar mammaplasty in association with a superior pedicle as the "premier" technique in breast reduction. As a trainee, I experienced both triumphs and defeats, successfully achieving large reductions, but then suffering through unexpected complications and aesthetic failures. Above all, I learned to manage the unexpected and seize every opportunity to optimize the outcome for the benefit of my patients.

I was honored to assist Madeleine Lejour performing her last breast reduction before retirement in October 1997. I watched in admiration as her amazing experience allowed her to remove over 1.5 kg of tissue per breast through the vertical scar technique she had made her own.

I am still convinced that there is no one "best" technique that can be applied to all breast reductions; rather, there are masters of some techniques based on enormous experience that can apply a particular technique to most cases, and then there are other cases that require different, more tailored techniques.

It was at this time that I began my quest to improve my technique in breast reduction. I spent much time and money attending specialist meetings and courses and visiting surgical colleagues. This enriched my global experience of breast surgery and opened my eyes and mind to new horizons and revolutionary concepts expounded upon by such luminaries as Hall-Findlay, Hammond, Würinger, and others.

By then I had relocated to Gent, where I could access the department's unassailable knowledge of and experience with perforator flaps and enhance my understanding of the blood supply to breast tissue. In this way I developed my own intellectually and clinically tried-and-tested breast reduction technique.

I would like to thank Dr. Madeleine Lejour for laying an invaluable foundation in vertical scar mammaplasty; Albert De Mey and Bruno Coessens, who took over in Brussels, and Dennis Goldschmidt for his boundless support. My deepest thanks go to Martyn Webster, my microsurgery mentor, a man who knew how to delegate responsibility and allowed me vast hands-on experience during my fellowship in Canniesburn-Glasgow. My heartfelt thanks and appreciation for all the support and encouragement extended to me by Professor Matton and my colleagues in the very special department in Gent. They have had the most profound influence on my career and my personal ideology: Koen, Stan, and Phillip, with you I have found my family again.

My personal appreciation to Foad Nahai and Dennis Hammond, my coeditors, for believing in me and accepting the responsibility for sharing this work. Thanks to Rozina and Petra for their help in preparing this book, to Kurt Drubbel of SiliconN imagE for his technical design and innovation, to Mr. Jef Van Tuerenhout for his colorful artistic paintings, and my gratitude to Irmela Bohn and Gabriele Schröder at Springer.

Finally, I would like to dedicate this book to the people without whom this endeavor would never have seen the light of day: my parents, my family, and my friends in Syria. To my daughter Sofie and to my wife Mirvat: a scientific career is very demanding and it steals time from the people whom we most love and care for.

Sofie, your daddy always misses you.

Mimi, the future is ours.

MOUSTAPHA HAMDI, MD, FCCP

Preface 2

The past decade has been witness to a paradigm shift in the treatment of macromastia and breast ptosis. With a blending of surgical techniques from every corner of the globe, the era of reduced scar breast surgery has arrived and is here to stay. These innovative techniques for breast reduction and mastopexy are applicable to almost any conceivable breast size or shape, provide consistent and reliable results that are maintained over time, and accomplish all this with roughly half the scar of older, more established approaches. This book details the various surgical techniques that allow this to be accomplished and draws on the experience of the finest breast surgeons in the world. Truly these times are academically and artistically a high-water mark in the history of breast surgery. My personal journey into this field has been influenced by many of the major contributors to the field of short scar breast surgery including Claude Lassus, Joca Sampaio Goes, Louis Bennelli, and Madeline Lejour. However, my greatest teachers have been Pat Maxwell and Jack Fisher. It was during my fellowship with these two fine surgeons that my artistic sensibilities were awakened and I discovered the courage to challenge conventional thinking. I developed the SPAIR mammaplasty drawing on the wisdom and expertise of those who came before me; however, I would be remiss if I did not recognize those who encouraged me and shared in our success as the procedure was developed. So to my wife Machelle and my children Rebecca, Sarah, and Andrew, who missed their husband and dad, all my love. To Joanie Bouwense, my nurse, first assistant, sounding board, and dear friend, my deepest thanks. To Mary McClain, who withstood the early struggles in the OR, my heartfelt appreciation. To John Beernink, MD, William Passinault, MD, Ron Ford, MD, and Carrie Bouwense, thank you for believing. It is my fervent hope that this book will allow every surgeon to embrace short scar breast surgery and achieve results never before seen. Our patients deserve nothing less. Good luck!

Dennis C. Hammond, MD

Preface 3

It has been a pleasure and a privilege to work with my coeditors Dr. Moustapha Hamdi and Dr. Dennis Hammond, as well as our contributors, to put together this truly international volume on short scar mammaplasty.

The term vertical refers only to the resultant scar and encompasses a number of operations, a variety of pedicles, and patterns of parenchymal resection, as well as differing methods of breast shaping. All of these leave the patient with better shape, more projection, and results that last over time. Our contributors have described their personal techniques encompassing these variables.

Why should we be concerned about scars? Many surgeons feel that as long as the breast has an aesthetic shape, scars are not important and that most patients with pleasing breast shape will not be concerned about the scars. We, however, feel that scars do matter, especially horizontal scars extending beyond the breast, past the anterior axillary line, and across the midline, misplaced horizontal scars that ride up above or below the preexisting crease onto the breast or abdomen. Scars do matter in younger women who may be more prone to hypertrophic scarring. Scars do matter to women who may be genetically predisposed to keloids. The ideal, of course, would be a pleasing breast shape with minimal scars. We feel that these short scar techniques offer both to our patients. I originally tried the short scar techniques in an effort to reduce scars. However, I have stayed with these techniques because I saw improved shape and results that have held up over time.

Short scar techniques have been popular in Europe and South America for a long time. Acceptance of the techniques in North America has been rather slow because of concerns over pedicle safety, learning curve, and, most of all, the perception that complications are more common with these techniques. In the chapter on complications, this myth is laid to rest and data are presented to demonstrate that the complication rate of these techniques is equal to or less than that with the standard Wise pattern techniques. Complications are related more to the patient's body mass index rather than technique. I believe that short scar techniques are here to stay and will continue to gain in popularity even in North America!

I would like to express my gratitude and indebtedness to those who have assisted me with the preparation of this book. I thank my partners and the fellows at Paces Plastic Surgery, my assistants Linda Neal and Tina Ruppert, my nurse Mary Popp, and our photographer Lester Robertson. They have all assisted me in every phase of the preparation of this book.

I also extend my gratitude to the staff at Springer, especially Irmela Bohn and Gabriele Schröder. Finally, let me express my thanks to my two coeditors, and especially to Dr. Moustapha Hamdi, who has done the lion's share of the work in putting this text together. Without his enthusiasm and efforts this volume would never have been completed.

FOAD NAHAI, MD, FACS

Vertical Mammaplasty: The Era of Maturity

MADELEINE LEJOUR

Breast reduction is one of the most difficult operations in plastic surgery because it should produce a beautiful, symmetrical, and durable result with minimal scarring. Raymond Vilain, the humorist of our profession, used to say that it takes 5 years to learn how to operate a breast properly...and 5 more years for the other. In addition, so many techniques are described that it is a real challenge to choose the best.

Twenty years ago vertical mammaplasty was practically unknown by most surgeons performing mastopexies and breast reductions. Devised by a French surgeon, Dartigues (1925), it was nearly forgotten until Arie (1957) and Lassus (1970) brought it to the attention of their colleagues. I admire Claude Lassus, a man with a vision who understood early that vertical mammaplasty not only reduced scarring but also produced better late results and that this justified the temporary strange appearance of the breasts.

Changes in our habits are difficult to make. I started using the technique in the late 1980s and was soon enthusiastic about the results. With the considerable experience accumulated by our team at the Department of Plastic Surgery of the University of Brussels, I had the opportunity to demonstrate and teach it in many meetings during the last decade of the century, adding my efforts to those of Lassus. Other surgeons who tried vertical mammaplasty contributed to the spread of the technique with a snowball effect, and I believe that all trainees in plastic surgery are now aware of its possibilities.

Changes in any technique are common, and most surgeons adapt operations for their personal practice. The changes aim for a better shape, a more durable result, and fewer complications. This requires a careful and honest evaluation of the results, which is not an easy task. First, recording all the data about the pre- and postoperative states of a patient is an endless fight for precision. Also, how do we explain major changes in the rate of complications when the technique is used in the same department during various periods? It may be that supervision of the residents was reduced if the team lacked trained surgeons for a period or that other, more impalpable factors intervened. Another example is the attention paid to certain data like obesity or preoperative volume of the breasts in the appreciation of complications. I was able to observe from my own experience that obesity per se increases the rate of complications and that the major factor of risk is a combination of obesity and very large breasts. All these major or minor factors explain why it is so difficult to obtain comparable evaluations. For a long time, evaluations were not even done. The rate of complications presented in publications was too vague to be taken into account. I am really very pleased to see that recent articles tend to better analyze and discuss complications. This is the best way to reduce them, improve the technique, and satisfy the patients who have placed their trust in us.

Development of our knowledge in areas other than surgical techniques deserves interest, for example, vascular anatomy in relation to surgery; breast content, which varies with menstrual cycle, parity, age, weight, and heredity; capacity for lactation, which combines hereditary and hormonal factors; variable fat degeneration after menopause; and so on. Let us hope that the interest will increase with time, just as it did for vertical mammaplasty.

A large number of presentations and publications in recent years have been devoted to vertical mammaplasty, and the time has come for an update of recent ideas, observations, technical modifications, and results. I do not doubt that the technique is now in its era of maturity and will survive the test of time.

Contents

Contributors

AFFONSO ACCORSI, Jr., MD
Plastic Surgeon, Rua Pereira Nunes,
Niteroi, RJ 24210-430, Rio de Janeiro, Brazil

PHILLIP BLONDEEL, MD, PhD
Professor, Plastic Surgery Department,
Gent University Hospital, Gent, Belgium

CLAUDIO CARDOSO DE CASTRO, MD
Professor and Chairman, Plastic Surgery Service,
University of the state of Rio de Janeiro,
Rua Carlos Goes, Rio de Janeiro, Brazil

SHEYLA MARIA CARVALHO RODRIGUES, MD
Plastic Surgeon,
Força Aérea do Galeão Hospital –
HFAG, Rio de Janeiro, Brazil

ELIZABETH J. HALL-FINDLAY, MD, FRCSC
Private practice, Mineral Springs Hospital,
Banff, Alberta, Canada

MOUSTAPHA HAMDI, MD, FCCP
Associate Professor, Gent University Hospital,
Plastic Surgery Department, Gent, Belgium

DENNIS C. HAMMOND, MD
Private practice, Center for Breast
and Body Contouring, Grand Rapids, MI, USA

M. KEITH HANNA, MD
Private Practice, Paces Plastic Surgery,
Atlanta, Georgia, USA

RAFIC KUZBARI, MD
Attendant Consultant in Plastic
and Reconstructive Surgery, Department
of Plastic Surgery, Wilhelminenspital,
Vienna, Austria

KOENRAAD VAN LANDUYT, MD, FCCP
Associate Professor, Gent University Hospital,
Plastic Surgery Department, Gent, Belgium

CLAUDE LASSUS, MD
Private practice, 1, Rue de Rivoli,
06000, Nice, France

ALBERT DE MEY, MD
Professor and Chairman,
Plastic Surgery Department, CHU-Brugmann,
Brussels, Belgium

STAN MONSTREY, MD, PhD
Professor and Chairman, Gent University Hospital,
Plastic Surgery Department, Gent, Belgium

FOAD NAHAI, MD, FACS
Private practice, Paces Plastic Surgery,
Atlanta, Georgia, USA, *and* Clinical Professor
of Plastic Surgery, Emory University,
Atlanta, Georgia, USA

LIACYR RIBEIRO, MD
Professor, Clinica Fluminense de Cirurgia Plastica,
Niteroi, Rio de Janeiro, Brazil

INGRID SCHLENZ, MD
Consultant Plastic Surgeon,
Department of Plastic Surgery,
Wilhelminenspital, Vienna, Austria

ELISABETH WUERINGER, MD
Consultant Plastic Surgeon, Department
of Plastic Surgery, Wilhelminenspital,
Vienna, Austria

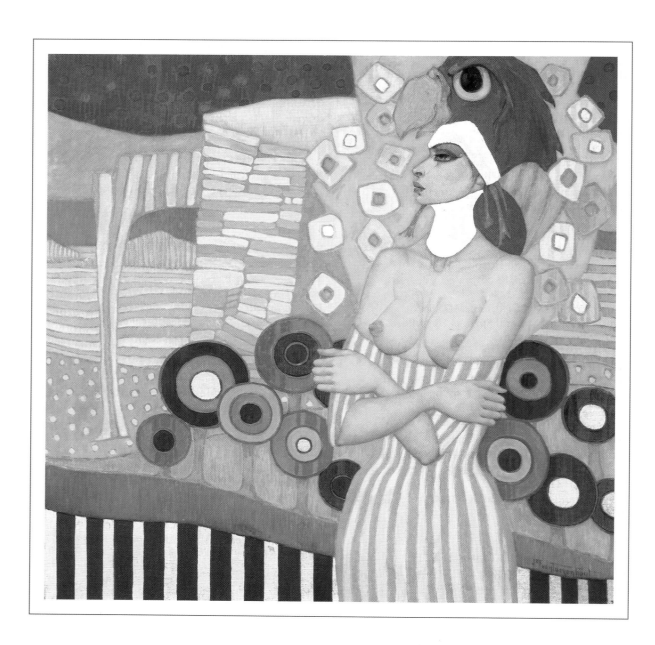

Anatomy of the Breast: A Clinical Application

MOUSTAPHA HAMDI, ELISABETH WÜRINGER, INGRID SCHLENZ, RAFIC KUZBARI

> The breast, by definition, is "the soft protuberant body adhering to the thorax in females, in which the milk is secreted for the nourishment of infants" or "the seat of affection and emotions; the repository of consciousness, designs and secrets...."
>
> *Merriam-Webster*

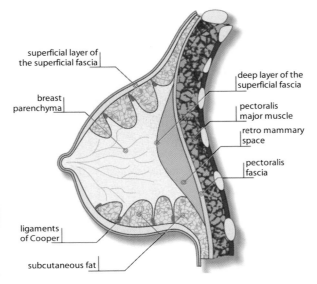

Fig. 1.1. Fascial system of the breast

General Anatomy

The epidermis of the nipple and areola is highly pigmented and somewhat wrinkled, and the skin of the nipple contains numerous sebaceous and apocrine sweat glands and relatively little hair. The 15 to 25 milk ducts enter the base of the nipple, where they dilate to form the milk sinuses. Slightly below the nipple's surface, these sinuses terminate in cone-shaped ampullae. The circular areola surrounds the nipple and varies between 15 and 60 mm in diameter. Its skin contains lanugo hair, sweat glands, sebaceous glands, and Montgomery's glands, which are large, modified sebaceous glands with miniature milk ducts that open into Morgagni's tubercles in the epidermis of the areola. Deep in the areola and nipple, bundles of smooth muscle fibers are arranged radially and circularly in the dense connective tissue and longitudinally along the lactiferous ducts that extend up into the nipple. These muscle fibers are responsible for the contraction of the areola, nipple erection, and emptying of the milk sinuses.

The majority of the breast parenchyma extends inferiorly from the level of the second or third rib to the inframammary fold, which is at about the level of the sixth or seventh rib, and laterally from the edge of the sternum to the anterior axillary line. The mammary tissue also extends variably into the axilla as the glandular Tail of Spence. The posterior surface of the breast rests on portions of the fasciae of the pectoralis major, serratus anterior, external abdominal oblique, and rectus abdominis muscles.

Fascial and Ligamentous System (Fig. 1.1)

The mammary tissue is enveloped by the superficial fascia of the anterior thoracic wall, which continuous above with the cervical fascia and below with the superficial abdominal fascia of Camper. The superficial layer of this fascia is poorly developed, especially in the upper part of the breast. It is an indistinct fibrous-fatty layer that is connected to, but separate from, dermis and breast tissue. This superficial fascial layer can be used effectively for suspension of the high-tension wound repair of breast-contouring procedures as described by Lockwood. The deep layer is better developed, lying in part on the pectoralis fascia. Between these two fasciae is the retromammary space filled with loose tissue that allows the breast to move freely over the chest wall. Projections of the deep layer of the superficial fascia cross this retromammary space, fuse with the pectoralis fascia, and form the posterior suspensory ligaments of the breast. The breast parenchyma may accompany these fibrous processes into the pectoralis major muscle itself. Therefore, complete removal of the breast parenchyma necessitates excision

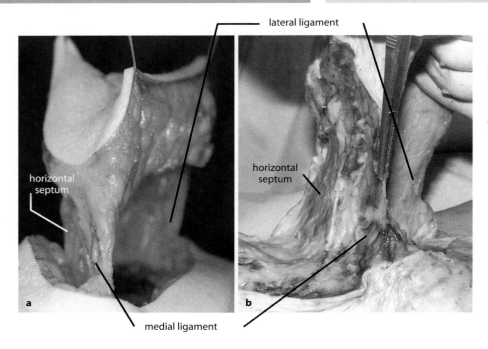

Fig. 1.2. **a** The ligamentous suspension in anatomical dissection of the right breast seen from cranio-medial [21]. **b** Equal preparation after intraarterial injection of surgical ink into internal thoracic artery [27]

of the pectoralis fascia and a layer of muscle as well. The superficial layer and skin are linked to the deep layer by the ligaments of Cooper, which are fibrous and elastic prolongations that divide the gland into multiple septa and give suspensory support to the breast. The breast parenchyma is made up of 15 to 25 lobes of glandular tissue, each emptying into a separate milk duct terminating in the nipple.

Horizontal Septum and Ligamentous Structures

The ligamentous suspension is a regularly situated fibrous structure that acts as a guiding structure for the main nerves and vessels to the breast and nipple-areola complex. The ligamentous suspension is comprised of a horizontal septum, originating at the pectoralis fascia along the fifth rib, bending upward into vertical ligaments at its medial and lateral border (Fig. 1.2). Cranially, and in an anterior direction, the vertical ligaments merge into the superficial fascia. The line of fixation of this ligamentous circle follows the borders of pectoralis major to a great extent. The horizontal septum is largely attached to the costal origin of pectoralis major along the fifth rib. The vertical ligaments follow the medial and lateral border of the muscle, and the cranial attachment of the superficial fascia corresponds to the deltopectoral groove. The ligamentous suspension can be found equally in female and male breasts.

The horizontal fibrous septum is a thin lamina of dense connective tissue that emerges from the pectoralis fascia at the level of the fifth rib and, traversing the breast from medial to lateral, extends to the middle of the nipple. It thereby divides the gland into a cranial and a caudal part. While heading to the nipple, it also divides the lactiferous ducts, emptying into the lactiferous sinuses, horizontally into two even planes of duct openings into the nipple. Thus the horizontal septum separates two anatomical units of glandular tissue (Fig. 1.3). The separation of the glandular tissue follows certain proportions insofar as the various volumes in different-sized breasts seem to be caused mainly by the cranial parenchymal layer of the horizontal septum. The cranial glandular layer in breasts of different size ranges from about 2 to about 7 cm, while the caudal glandular layer always has a constant thickness of about 2 cm. Clinically, the horizontal septum can thus act as a useful guide for achieving symmetry in breast reductions.

At its medial and lateral borders the horizontal septum becomes even denser and curves upward into vertically directed ligaments. The medial vertical ligament is a strong structure that originates from the sternum at the level of the second to the fifth rib. The lateral vertical ligament is a rather weak fibrous structure that emerges from the pectoralis fascia at the lateral edge of pectoralis minor. The horizontal septum and its vertical extensions thereby build constantly a sling of dense connective tissue that connects the gland

Fig. 1.3. **a** The horizontal fibrous septum seen from medially in anatomical dissection of left breast divides the breast into a cranial and a caudal glandular layer [23]. **b** Same view in schematic diagram [21]. **c** Cranial vascular layer seen from cranially in anatomical dissection after intraarterial injection of surgical ink into thoracoacromial artery [27]

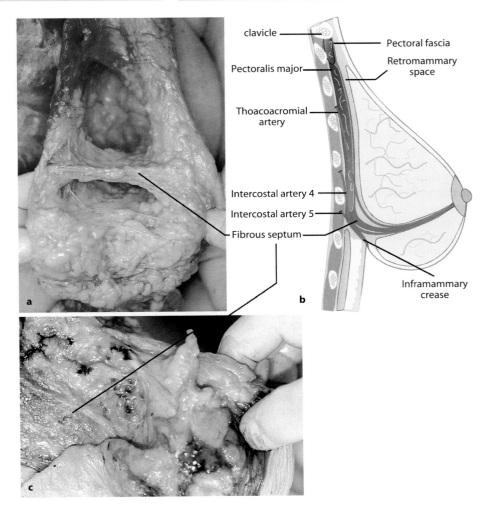

Fig. 1.4. Anterior view of left breast in schematic diagram showing the superficial (*yellow*) and the deep part (*gray*) of the ligamentous suspension

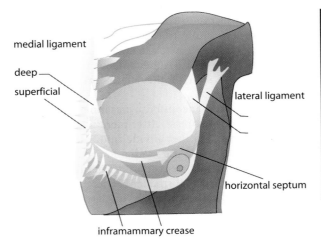

Fig. 1.5. Ligamentous suspension in anatomical preparation of right breast, cranial view

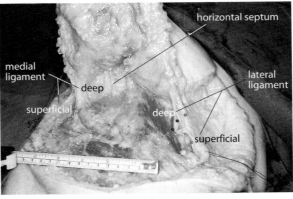

to the thoracic wall (Fig. 1.4). This is the deep part of the ligamentous suspension, which guides the neurovascular supply to the nipple, similar to the mesentery of the intestine. The remaining parts of the breast receive no distinct vessels from the thoracic wall.

This suspensory circle of connective tissue also has a superficial part that inserts into the skin medially, caudally, and laterally, thereby defining the extent the borders of the breast (Figs. 1.4 and 1.5). The medial superficial ligament is rather weak and extends from the deep medial ligament into the overlying skin. The firm lateral superficial ligament has a strong suspensory function that it fulfills by attaching the deep lateral ligament to the axillary fascia along the midaxillary line. It produces the concavity of the armpit and thus corresponds to the suspensory ligament of the axilla. The origin of the horizontal septum from the pectoralis fascia along the fifth rib carries the weight of the breast and prevents descending of the base of the breast. A densification of Cooper's ligaments from the origin of the horizontal septum into the inframammary crease skin represents its superficial part.

The vertical ligaments merge into the superficial mammary fascia in a cranial and in an anterior direction. Thus, the ligamentous suspension also connects with the ligamenta suspensoria, described as stretching from the mammary fascia into the skin [1]. The ligamentous suspension provides sturdy fibrous structures that can be used for modeling and fixation of the gland intraoperatively, in contrast to the residual breast parenchyme, where sutures tend to cut through the tissues.

The ligamentous suspension can easily be accessed clinically, which allows for locating and maintaining the main neurovascular supply intraoperatively. The horizontal septum can be found by following the retromammary space bluntly in a caudal direction to the level of the fourth intercostal space (Fig. 1.3). Here, the retromammary space changes direction and continues as a loose areolar tissue plane that heads horizontally to the nipple. Below this easily created cleavage plane an even plane of vessels gets faintly through, which builds the cranial vascular layer. This vascular layer is caudally attached to the horizontal septum. By gentle, blunt finger dissection, the horizontal areolar plane can be progressively opened up, thereby leaving the neurovascular supply intact. The areolar plane can be followed to the nipple, which is also divided horizontally by the horizontal septum, and it may, indeed, become less distinct as it approaches the nipple (Fig. 1.3). The vertical ligaments can also be accessed by blunt dissection along the retromammary space. When following the lateral rim of the horizontal septum bluntly, the later-

al ligament is encountered. The medial ligament delineates the retromammary space in a medial direction.

Innervation of the Breast

In the past, the innervation of the breast received little attention in anatomic textbooks, and published reports were contradictory concerning the distribution and course of the supplying nerves. The British surgeon Sir Astley Cooper was one of the first to investigate the innervation of the breast 135 years ago, and some of his findings are still valid today. Ever since, authors have agreed that the skin of the breast and the gland is innervated by the lateral and anterior branches of the intercostal nerves; however, there is wide disagreement about which intercostal nerves are involved.

In a recent study (Schlenz et al. 2000) we determined the origin and course of the nerves supplying the breast and the nipple-areola complex.

Innervation of the Gland and the Breast Skin

The breast is innervated by the lateral and anterior cutaneous branches of the second to sixth intercostal nerves. The lateral cutaneous branches pierce the intercostal muscles and the deep fascia in the midaxillary line and take an inferomedial course. The second lateral cutaneous branch terminates in the axillary tail of the breast. The third, fourth, fifth, and sixth lateral cutaneous branches continue on the surface of the serratus anterior for 3–5 cm. At the border of the pectoral muscle they divide into a deep and a superficial branch. The deep branch courses below or within the pectoral fascia to the midclavicular line, where it turns for almost 90° to run through the gland, giving off several branches (Figs. 1.6 and 1.7). The superficial branch runs in the subcutaneous tissue and terminates in the skin of the lateral breast (Figs. 1.6 and 1.7).

The anterior cutaneous branches innervate the medial portion of the breast. After piercing the fascia in the parasternal line they divide into a lateral and a medial branch. While the medial branch crosses the lateral border of the sternum, the lateral branch divides again into several smaller branches, which take an inferolateral course through the subcutaneous tissue. They become progressively more superficial along their way and terminate in the breast skin or at the areolar edge (Figs. 1.6 and 1.8). The supraclavicular nerves terminate in the skin of the superior part of the breast.

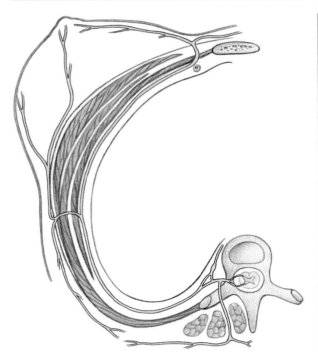

Fig. 1.6. Schematic drawing of breast and anterior (ACB) and lateral cutaneous branches (LCB) of fourth intercostal nerve innervating the nipple and areola. (Reprinted with permission from Lippincott, Williams and Wilkins: Plast Reconstr Surg 105:905, 2000)

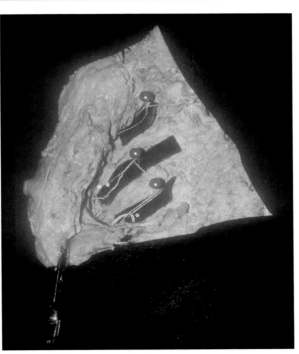

Fig. 1.7. Lateral view of a left breast (*double asterisk*: lateral cutaneous branch of the fourth intercostal nerve reaching the posterior surface of the nipple; *asterisk*: cutaneous divisions of the lateral cutaneous branches terminating in the skin and gland of the lateral breast)

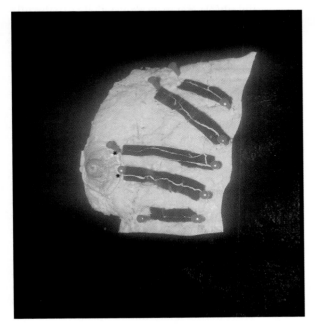

Fig. 1.8. Anterior view of a right breast: *asterisks*: third and fourth anterior cutaneous branch terminating at the medial border of the areola (Reprinted with permission from Lippincott, Williams and Wilkins: Plast Reconstr Surg 105:905, 2000)

Innervation of the Nipple and Areola

The innervation of the nipple and areola shows frequent variations in the course and distribution of the supplying nerves, which explains the controversial findings of previous studies. The nipple and areola are always innervated by both the anterior and lateral cutaneous branches of the third, fourth, or fifth intercostal nerves. But the number, distribution, and size of these nerves vary: the more numerous the nerves, the smaller are their diameters.

Lateral Cutaneous Branches (Table 1.1)

The fourth lateral cutaneous branch is the most constant nerve to the nipple – it supplies the nipple in 93% of breasts. In 79% of breasts it is the only lateral nerve to the nipple. Other possible patterns of nerve supply to the nipple are summarized in Table 1.1. The two lateral cutaneous branches of the third and fourth intercostal nerves can also form an anastomosis lateral to the border of the pectoral muscle and supply the nipple with the resulting single nerve branch. Another possibility is the division of the lateral cutaneous

Table 1.1. Innervation of the nipple-areola complex; *ICN*, intercostal nerve

Lateral cutaneous branches of ICN		Anterior cutaneous branches of ICN	
3rd	3.5%	3rd	21.4%
4th	79.0%	4th	7.1%
5th	3.5%	3rd and 4th	57.1%
3rd, 4th	7.0%	4th and 5th	10.7%
4th, 5th	7.0%	3rd, 4th, and 5th	3.5%

branch of the fourth intercostal nerve into two smaller branches, both of which reach the posterior surface of the nipple within a short distance of each other.

In 93% of breasts, the deep branches of the lateral cutaneous nerves innervate the nipple, running below or within the pectoral fascia. On reaching the midclavicular line they turn almost 90° and continue through the glandular tissue toward the posterior surface of the nipple, which they enter with several tiny branches (Figs. 1.6 and 1.7). In 7% of breasts the superficial branch of the lateral cutaneous nerves innervates the nipple. These nerves run in the subcutaneous tissue close to the skin and reach the nipple from the lateral side.

Anterior Cutaneous Branches (Table 1.1)

The anterior cutaneous branches contribute to the medial innervation of the nipple-areola complex. The branches that terminate at the areolar edge originate from the third, fourth, or fifth intercostal nerves. They always reach the areolar edge between the 8 and 11 o'clock position in the left breast and between the 1 and 4 o'clock position in the right breast (Figs. 1.6 and 1.8). Innervation can derive from the third and fourth anterior cutaneous branches (57.1%).

The innervation of the nipple and areola is very complex due to frequent variations of the course and distribution of the supplying nerves. The most common innervation pattern is a lateral innervation by the fourth lateral cutaneous branch, which takes a "deep" course within the pectoralis fascia and reaches the nipple from its posterior surface, and a medial innervation by the third and fourth anterior cutaneous branches, which take a "superficial" course within the subcutaneous tissue and reach the medial areolar edge. These nerves are best protected if surgical resection at the base of the breast and skin incisions at the medial edge of the areola are avoided. Studies on nipple sensitivity before and after reduction mammaplasty indicate a better preservation of sensitivity after inferior pedicle techniques in comparison to superior pedicle techniques and are in keeping with these findings. However, since variations are possible, breast surgery is still associated with the risk of impairing the sensitivity of the nipple and areola.

Blood Supply of the Breast

Arterial System

Three main arterial routes supply the breast: the internal mammary artery, the lateral thoracic artery, and the intercostal arteries (Fig. 1.9).

1. The internal mammary artery, a branch of the subclavian artery, provides approximately 60% of total breast flow, mainly to the medial portion, by anterior and posterior perforating branches (Fig. 1.10). The anterior perforating branches exit their respective intercostal spaces approximately 2 cm laterally to the sternum. The second and third anterior perforating branches are by far the most significant. The first and fourth are less constant. These branches run within the subcutaneous tissue of the breast and may be found 0.5 to 1 cm from the medial surface of the skin. They course inferiorly and laterally to anastomose with branches of the lateral thoracic artery at the nipple. Anastomoses with the intercostal arteries occur less frequently. The posterior perforating branches exit more laterally from the intercostal spaces and supply the posterior aspect of the breast.

2. The lateral thoracic artery arises from the axillary artery or, rarely, from the thoracoacromial or subscapular artery. This artery supplies up to 30% of breast blood flow to the lateral and upper outer portions of the breast. The branches course inferomedially within the subcutaneous tissue to effect anastomoses with branches of the internal mammary and intercostal arteries in the areolar area. Because there is often more subcutaneous tissue laterally than medially, they are frequently found from 1 to 2.5 cm from the skin surface. As the areola is approached, all of these vessels become more superficial.

3. The third, fourth, and fifth posterior intercostal arteries are the least important of the arteries supplying the breast. Originating from the aorta, they course in the intercostal spaces and mainly supply the inferoexternal quadrant of the breast. Additional minor sources of arterial supply to the breast include branches from the axillary artery, the thoracic artery, the subscapular artery, and the pectoral branches of the thoracoacromial artery.

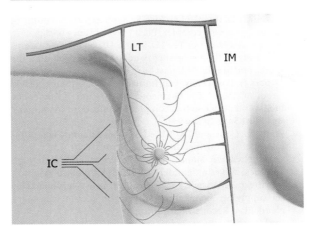

Fig. 1.9. Three main arterial routes supplying the breast: internal mammary artery (IM), lateral thoracic (LT) artery, and intercostal (IC) arteries

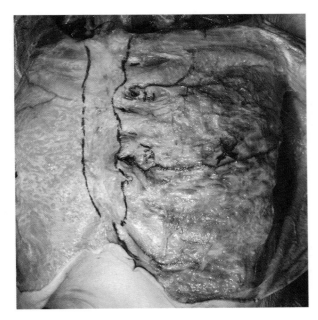

Fig. 1.10. Injection study on cadavers shows communicating branches of IM and LT vessels, which run in the subcutaneous tissue provide the main blood supply to the nipple-areola complex (*cross*)

The Venous Drainage

The venous drainage of the breast is divided into a superficial system and a deep system.

1. The superficial system lies just below the superficial layer of the superficial fascia and has been classified into two main types: transverse and longitudinal. The transverse veins (91%) run medially in the subcutaneous tissues and join perforating vessels that empty into the internal mammary vein. Longitudinal vessels (9%) ascend to the suprasternal notch and empty into the superficial veins of the lower neck.

2. Three groups of veins are involved in the deep drainage system of the breast:
   (a) Perforating branches of the internal mammary vein, which are the largest vessels of the deep system and empty into the corresponding innominate veins.
   (b) Tributaries of the axillary vein.
   (c) Perforating branches of posterior inercostal veins. These veins communicate with the vertebral veins and the azygos vein, which leads to the superior vena cava.

All three of these venous pathways lead to the pulmonary capillary network and provide a route for metastatic carcinoma emboli to the lungs. The vertebral system of veins provides an entirely different metastatic route. These veins form a vertebral venous plexus and provide a direct venous pathway for metastases to bones of the spine, pelvis, femur, shoulder girdle, humerus, and skull.

Blood Supply of the Nipple-Areola Complex

The main blood supply to the nipple-areola complex is provided by branches of the internal mammary and lateral thoracic artery, which run in the subcutaneous tissue and communicate with each other above and below the areola. Small branches derived from the communicating vessels were found running toward the nipple-areola complex (Fig. 1.10). These small vessels reach the base of the nipple, giving off fine vessels to the areolar skin, and ascend into the nipple in a circular fashion. These ascending vessels arborize in the upper and middle thirds of the nipple.

The periareolar dermal and subdermal plexus, which provide the anatomic base for preserving the nipple-areola complex in reduction mammaplasties, were found not to be particularly vascular and not to anastomose widely with the plexus in the nipple-areola complex. A medial or a lateral glandular pedicle provides the best blood supply to the nipple-areola complex by including these communicating branches within the subcutaneous tissue. A pure central pedicle must be wide enough to incorporate enough fine vessels of the thoracacromial artery to provide adequate blood supply. A superior pedicle should be large enough to include subdermal connections to the lateral and medial communication vessels. In the inferior pedicle, the blood supply comes from cutaneous perforators of the fourth and/or fifth intercostal arteries, which are usually large.

References

1. Cooper AP (1840) On the Anatomy of the Breast. Longman, Orme, Green, Brown and Longmans, London
2. Eckhard C (1851) Die Nerven der weiblichen Brustdrüse und ihr Einfluß auf die Milchsekretion. Beitr Anat Physiol 1:1–9
3. Addison C (1905) Ellis's Demonstrations of Anatomy, 12th edn. Smith Elder, London
4. Hamilton WJ (1966) Textbook of human anatomy, 2nd edn. Mcmillan, London
5. Woodbourne RT, Burkel WE (1994) Essentials of Human Anatomy, 9th edn. Oxford University Press, Oxford, UK
6. Brash JC, Jamieson EB (ed) (1943) Cunningham's Textbook of Anatomy, 8th edn. Oxford University Press, London
7. Maliniac JW (1943) Arterial blood supply of the breast. Arch Surg 47:329
8. Maliniac JW (1950) Breast Deformities and Their Repair. Grune and Stratton, New York, pp 14
9. Massopust LC, Gardner WD (1950) Infrared photographic studies of the superficial thoracic veins in the female. Surg Gynecol Obstet 91:717
10. Craig RD, Sykes PA (1970) Nipple sensitivity following reduction mammaplasty. Br J Plast Surg 23:165
11. Edwards EA (1976) Surgical anatomy of the breast. In: Goldwyn RM (ed) Plastic and Reconstructive Surgery of the Breast. Little, Brown, Boston
12. Serafin D (1976) Anatomy of the breast. In: Georgiade NG (ed) Reconstructive Breast Surgery. Mosby, St Louis, p 18
13. Farina MA, Newby BG, Alani HM (1980) Innervation of the nipple-areola complex. Plast Reconstr Surg 66:497
14. Haagensen CD (1986) Anatomy of the mammary glands. In: Haagensen CD (ed) Diseases of the Breast, 3rd edn. Saunders, Philadelphia
15. Williams PL, Warwick R, Dyson M, Bannister LH (eds) (1989) Gray's Anatomy, 37th edn. Churchill Livingstone, Edinburgh, UK
16. Sandsmark M, Amland PF, Abyholm F, Traaholt L (1992) Reduction mammaplasty: a comparative study of the Orlando and Robbins methods in 292 patients. Scand J Plast Reconstr Hand Surg 26:203
17. Nakajima H, Imanishi N, Aiso S (1995) Arterial anatomy of the nipple-areola complex. Plast Reconstr Surg 96:843
18. Sarhadi NS, Dunn JS, Lee FD, Soutar DS (1996) An anatomical study of the nerve supply of the breast, including the nipple and areola. Br J Plast Surg 49:156
19. Jaspars JJ, Posma AN, van Immerseel AA, Gittenberger-de Groot AC (1997) The cutaneous innervation of the female breast and nipple-areola complex: implications for surgery. Br J Plast Surg 50:249
20. Bland KI, Copeland EM III (eds) (1998) Anatomy and physiology of the normal and lactating breast. In: The Breast: Comprehensive Management of Benign and Malignant Diseases, 2nd edn. Saunders, Philadelphia, vol 1, p 19
21. Würinger E, Mader N, Posch E, Holle J (1998) Nerve and vessel supplying ligamentous suspension of the mammary gland. Plast Reconstr Surg 101:1486
22. Lockwood T (1999) Reduction mammaplasty and mastopexy with superficial fascial system suspension. Plast Reconstr Surg 103:1411
23. Würinger E (1999) Refinement of the central pedicle breast reduction by application of the ligamentous suspension. Plast Reconstr Surg 103:1400
24. Hamdi M, Greuse M, DeMey A, Webster MHC (1999) Breast sensation after superior pedicle versus inferior pedicle mammaplasty: prospective clinical evaluation. Br J Plast Surg 54:39
25. Schlenz I, Kuzbari R, Gruber H, Holle J (2000) The sensitivity of the nipple-areola complex: an anatomic study. Plast Reconstr Surg 105:905
26. Hamdi M, Greuse M, Nemec E, Deprez C, DeMey A (2001) Breast sensation after superior pedicle versus inferior pedicle mammaplasty: anatomical and histological evaluation. Br J Plast Surg 54:43
27. Wueringer E, Tschabitscher M (2003) New aspects of the topography of the mammary gland regarding its neurovascular supply along a regular ligamentous suspension. Eur J Morphol 40(3):181
28. Hamdi M, Van de Sijpe K, Van Landuyt K, Blondeel PN, Monstrey S (2003) Evaluation of nipple-areola complex sensitivity after the latero-central glandular pedicle technique in breast reduction. Br J Plast Surg 56:360

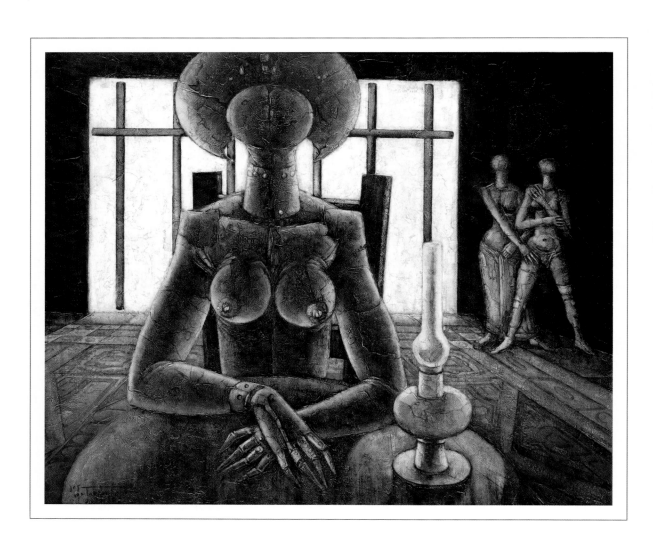

Long-Lasting Results of Vertical Mammaplasty

CLAUDE LASSUS

 he breast will feed the baby and will delight the father.

This sentence from the Koran summarizes the two main functions of the breast:

- Feeding
- Sexual symbol

It is obvious that any type of surgery on the breasts must protect those two functions. This is why, to me, safety is first; shape is second in mammaplasty.

Achieving beautiful and long-lasting results in a safe way is mandatory in breast reduction.

Claude Lassus

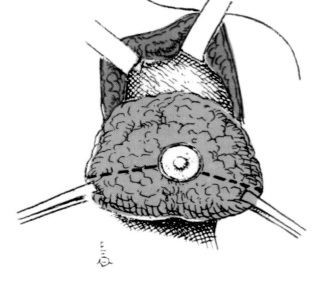

Fig. 3.1. Aubert's technique

Introduction

Aubert, a French surgeon from Marseille, described in 1923 what is supposed to be the first tru mammaplasty [1]. When I say true mammaplasty, this means that for the first time a surgeon proposed a technique allowing him not only to reduce the size of the breast but also to relocate the nipple-areola complex. Looking at the drawings of the Aubert technique (Fig. 3.1), we notice that this surgeon undermined the skin widely from the gland and the gland from the muscle.

These principles were used in almost all the techniques that followed and of course in the Biesenberger procedure, which was the most popular mammaplasty between the 1930s and the 1980s [2]. Meanwhile, complications were many: seromas, haematomas, infections, skin necrosis, fat necrosis, glandular necrosis, and nipple-areola necrosis. Another problem was that, after months and even years, there was an important bottoming out of the breast, producing a typical *"clog aspect"* (*"Sein en Sabot"*). So in the Biesenberger technique complications were fre-

quent and results not long lasting. Why? Because of the principles of the technique I have already mentioned: skin and gland undermining.

In the 1960s, Pitanguy et al. [3–5] brought new principles that made mammaplasty a safer operation with better results. The principles are the following:
- Resection "en bloc"
- No or less undermining
- Transposition of the nipple areola on dermoglandular flaps.

Since then, mammaplasty has been *a safer operation*. Safety is one of the goals of this operation; the other goals are:
- A good reduction of the size of the breast
- A minimal scar to finish off
- A beautiful and long-lasting result

Beautiful results are obtained now with many procedures, but long-lasting results remain a challenge. What are the keys to obtaining a breast that remains beautiful in the long term?

First Key: No Skin or Gland Undermining

The first question is: What causes bottoming out? Gravity, of course, seems to be the simple answer. However, we must consider some anatomic features.

The mammary gland is enclosed between the superficial and deep layers of the superficial fascia. The deep layer splits off the superficial fascia and passes deep to the mammary gland. Between the deep layer and the fascia of the pectoralis major is a well-defined space: the retromammary space. The retromammary space contains loose areolar tissue and allows the breast to glide freely over the chest wall. Portions of the deep layer of the superficial fascia form connective tissue extensions that pass through the retromammary space and join with the fascia of the pectoralis major. These extensions help support the breast, but the mammary gland is more intimately connected with the skin than with the muscle. Particularly in the young, the adherent elastic skin and its subcutaneous structures play a dominant supportive role.

The skin of the breast is closely adherent to the underlying structures. It serves to support the organ both by its elasticity and by virtue of the fibrous connections between it and the gland. Numerous strong fibrous projections extend into the inner aspect of the skin covering. These processes constitute the ligamenta suspensoria or Cooper's ligaments (Fig. 3.2). They link the skin to the gland, the gland to the nipple, and the various portions of the gland to one another. Once the skin and its suspensory ligaments are stretched and weakened, they do not regain their supportive ability. So bottoming out can be caused by:

- Poor skin tone, stretch marks, skin damaged by sun or corticosteroid therapy, etc.
- Or by the fact that Cooper's ligaments have been stretched and weakened by:
  - Repeated lactations
  - Repeated variations of weight
  - Strain imposed by mammary hypertrophy
  - Deflation-producing glandular involution

As early as 1970 [6], I established that skin and gland did not have to be elevated. I still strongly believe that skin undermining is a mistake. We must preserve the integrity of Cooper's ligaments to help produce long-lasting results.

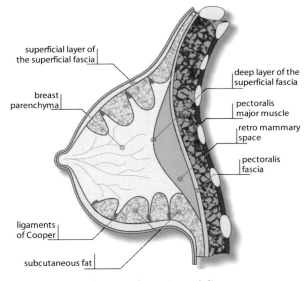

Fig. 3.2. A sagittal section shows Cooper's ligaments

Second Key: A Central Vertical Wedge Resection

We must produce a **beautiful breast**. It is common to hear "Don't compromise the shape for a short scar." Figure 3.3 shows the result of a mammaplasty performed by a board-certified plastic surgeon. We notice the following:

- A flat upper pole
- An upward-looking nipple areola due to the bottoming out of the breast
- A classic long inverted T scar

This demonstrates:

- A long scar does not guarantee a beautiful result.
- The scar plays no role in achieving a good result.
  To reduce the size of a breast, we can use:

A horizontal resection. In this type of resection, the hypertrophic ptotic portion of the breast is removed at the level of the inframammary fold. When this has been achieved, only the portion of the breast located above the fold remains: this portion is flat, which is why the new breast will be flat.

A vertical resection. Pinching the inferior midbreast with the fingers gives projection to the breast and fullness at the upper pole. The same can be obtained by removing the inferior midpart of the breast through a wedge resection. After that we bring together the lateral edges of the remaining breast (Fig. 3.4 a–c).

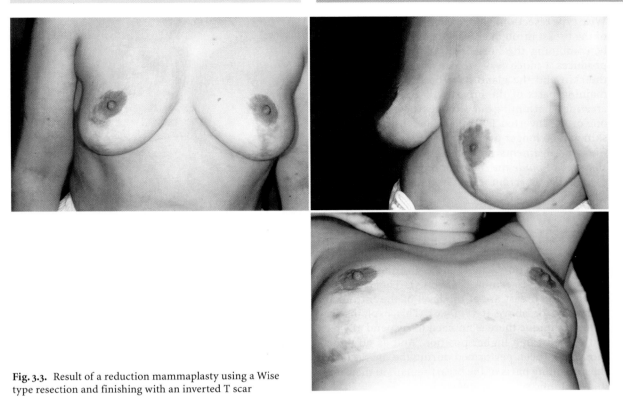

Fig. 3.3. Result of a reduction mammaplasty using a Wise type resection and finishing with an inverted T scar

Fig. 3.4a–c. Comparing pre-operative markings between Lejour's (*green*) and Lasuss's techniques (*violet*): there is no mosque dome and the junction of the vertical lines is higher above the inframammary fold in Lassus's drawing compared to this one by Lejour. The superior pedicle flap is the same in both techniques

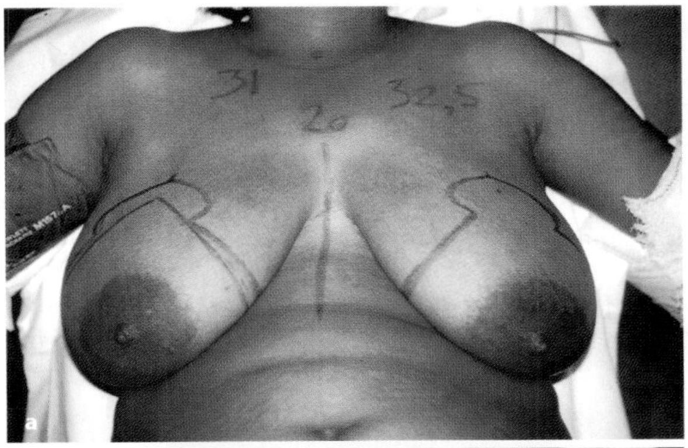

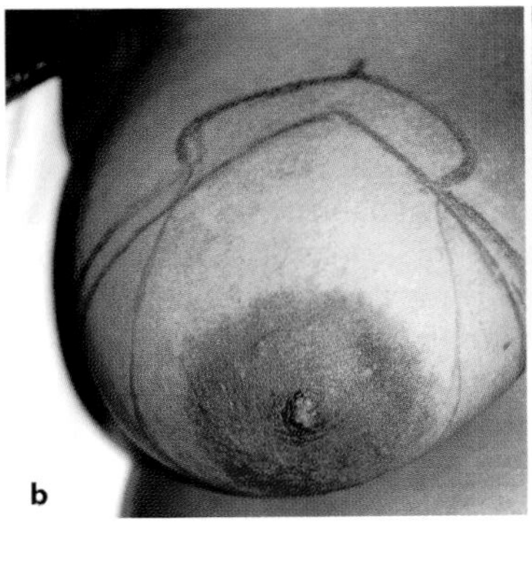

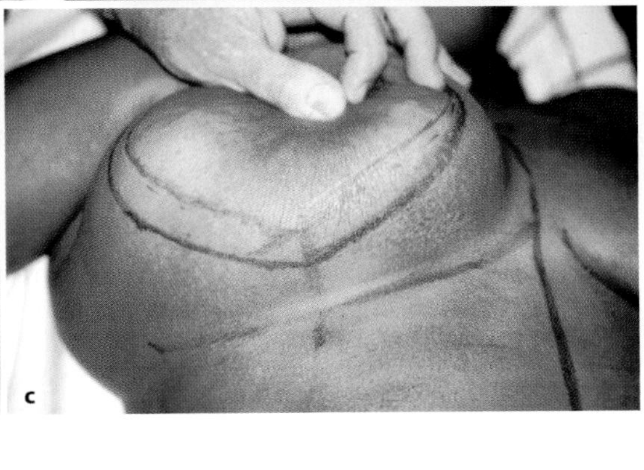

Wise type resection.   Most techniques reduce the size of the breast through a Wise type resection. Obviously, combining the horizontal and vertical resection produces a much less projected breast. Moreover, if the skin and the gland have been detached, the remaining parts of the breast will glide and descend, creating a bottoming out, whether the scar is a vertical one or an "inverted T." This is due to the fact that the skin will no longer play a supportive role because the Cooper's ligaments have been severed. *This is why since 1964 I made the choice of the central vertical "en bloc" wedge resection without skin and glandular undermining.*

Third Key: A Central Vertical Wedge Resection

With this resection almost the entire ptotic portion of the breast is removed (Fig. 3.5). The remaining parts of the breast are at the level of the inframammary fold or above it (Fig. 3.6). This explains why in my technique there is no need to suspend any part of the breast in a higher position. And as no undermining has been performed during the operation, all the remaining parts of the breast remain in their original anatomic situation and structure.

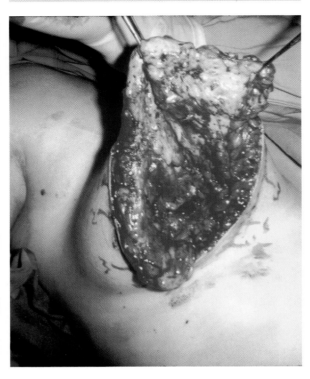

Fig. 3.6. The central vertical wedge resection is performed

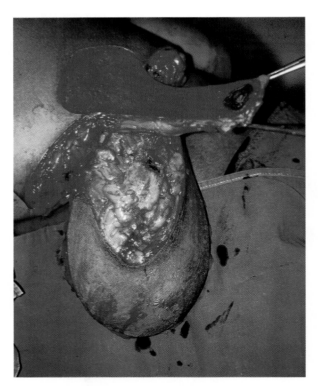

Fig. 3.5. The superior pedicle flap is elevated in preparation for the central wedge resection

Fourth Key: The Vertical Scar

With the central vertical wedge resection the breast cone is reconstructed by drawing the lateral parts of the remaining breast centrally toward each other. This maneuver eliminates almost any dead space in the breast, and overall it puts in close contact two composite blocks made of skin, fat, and gland. These two blocks are congruent: they fit perfectly. There is no need to cheat with the skin (Fig. 3.7). They are maintained in close contact by a row of inverted stitches of a permanent material that catches the deep dermis (Fig. 3.8).

I don't believe stitches should be used for catching the tissues underneath the deep dermis. Most of the time the tissue in this area consists of fat rather than gland and stitches do not have long-lasting action. At any rate, the healing that occurs produces a strong vertical fibrous band, which plays the same role as the whalebone in a corset. This, it seems to me, is another reason why my vertical technique produces long-lasting results (Figs. 3.9–3.11).

In summary, my technique produces long-lasting results for four reasons:
- No skin or glandular undermining: This allows the skin to keep its supportive role to the organ.

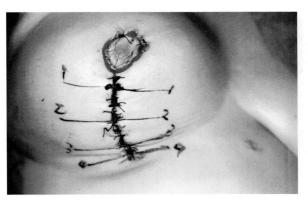

Fig. 3.7. Two congruent composite blocks are stitched together

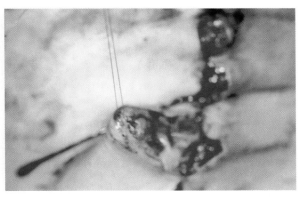

Fig. 3.8. The deep dermis of the vertical incision is stitched tightly using nonabsorbable monofilament sutures

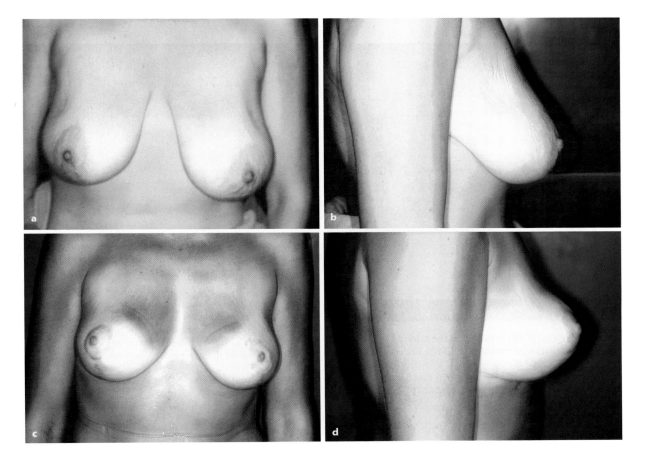

Fig. 3.9. a, b Before. c, d After, 5 years post-operatively

- A central vertical wedge resection: This type of resection gives fullness at the upper pole and projection to the breast.
- The central vertical wedge resection: This technique eliminates almost the entire ptotic portion of the breast, leaving the rest in its original position.

- The vertical suture: This produces a vertical band of fibrotic tissue that plays the role of a whalebone in a corset.

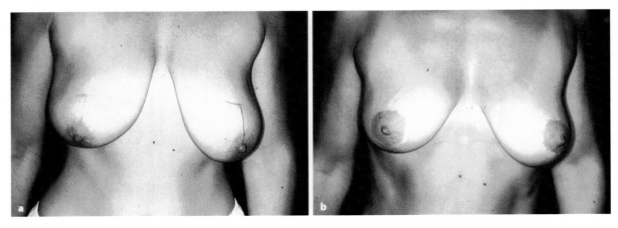

Fig. 3.10. **a** Before. **b** 10 years post-operatively (2 pregnancies meantime). Looking at the two naevi one can notice the good elevation of the breasts after 10 years and in spite of a poor quality of skin

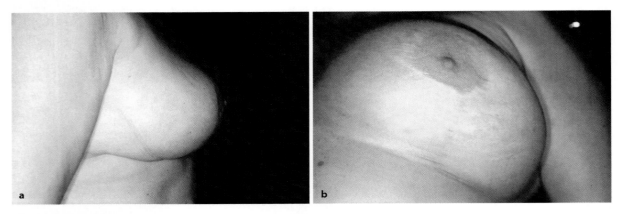

Fig. 3.11 a,b. Result 30 years postoperatively. **a** Projection ID still good. **b** Vertical scar is incon-spicuous

References

1. Aubert V (1923) Hypertrophie mammaire de la puberté – résection partielle restauratrice. Arch Franco-Belges Chir 3:284
2. Biesenberger H (1931) Deformitäten und Kosmetische Operationen der weiblichen Brust. Mandrich, Vienna
3. Pitanguy I (1960) Breast hypertrophy. In: Transactions of the International Society of Plastic Surgeons, 2nd Congress, London. Livingstone, Edinburgh, UK (1960), p 509
4. Strömbeck JO (1960) Mammaplasty: report of a new technique based on the two pedicles procedure. Br J Plast Surg 13:79
5. Skoog T (1963) A technique of breast resection. Acta Chir Scand 26:453
6. Lassus C (1970) A technique for breast reduction. Int Surg 53:69

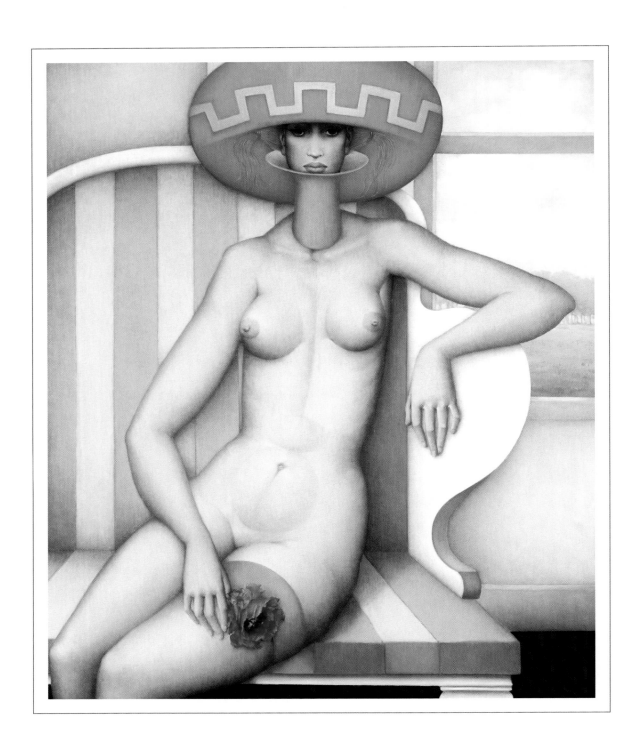

Incisions and Resection of Breast Tissue

Step 1. The first step is to make the medial, inferior, and lateral incisions through the skin and subcutaneous tissues. It is often possible to make this incision while the mammostat is still in place.

Step 2. Once the incision has been made, upward traction is placed on the breast and the inferior flap is elevated. Through the lower incision a thin 3- to 4-mm-thick flap is elevated from the lower incision down to the preexisting inframammary fold. Just above the level of the preexisting inframammary fold, this dissection extends onto the pectoralis fascia. I feel it is extremely important not to dissect below the preexisting fold in order to preserve it. This dissection is then extended for a variable distance medially and laterally to facilitate the resection of a small segment of tissue at the base of the medial and lateral pillars (Fig. 4.11).

Step 3. The medial dissection is then performed. The breast is pulled laterally so that the medial incision is in line with the vertical axis of the breast as marked on the abdominal wall (Fig. 4.12). The dissection continues straight through the breast tissue down to the pectoralis fascia. I prefer to do this with the cutting and coagulating electrocautery in order to minimize blood loss. Once the medial incision has been made, the breast is then pulled medially and the lateral dissection is made with the lateral line of dissection in line with the vertical axis (Fig. 4.13). This dissection also extends to the chest wall and pectoralis fascia. Every attempt should be made not to enter the pectoralis fascia or the muscle itself. This will not only reduce bleeding; it will also significantly reduce postoperative pain.

Step 4. With the completion of the medial and lateral dissection the breast tissue is elevated off the pectoralis fascia, leaving the fascia intact. On each side, inferiorly, a small triangular extension of breast tissue is included with the specimen. The dissection is continued from below upward under the existing nipple and up toward the new nipple position. I usually stop this dissection at the projected new nipple position. The bulk of the breast tissue to be resected has now been mobilized.

Step 5. The central and lower breast tissue is now separated from the deepithelialized superior pedicle, usually 2–3 cm below the areola margin (Fig. 4.14). In a short reduction, this dissection is continued at a 90° angle straight down to the chest wall and the specimen resected. With a large reduction and a long superior pedicle, the superior pedicle is thinned distally and the dissection continues upward to the level of the projected nipple and then down to the chest wall. The

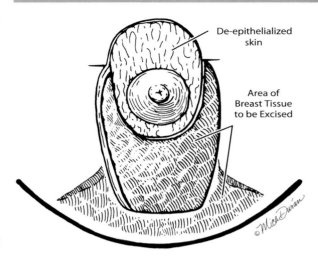

De-epithelialized skin

Area of Breast Tissue to be Excised

Fig. 4.11. The extent of the breast tissue to be resected

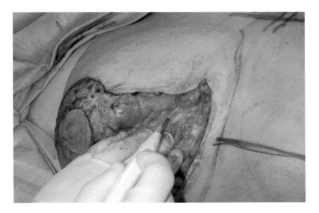

Fig. 4.12. The breast is retracted laterally, and the incision is made through the breast tissue to make the medial pillar

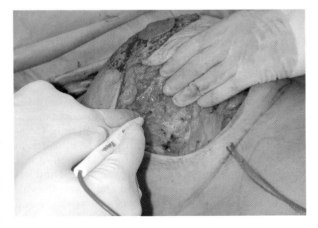

Fig. 4.13. The breast is displaced medially and the dissection made directly through the breast tissue toward the pectoralis to make the lateral pillar

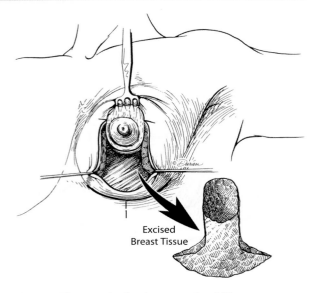

Fig. 4.14. The resection has been completed. The retractors are at the base of the medial and lateral pillars, and the resected specimen shows the small triangle of breast tissue resected above the inframammary fold on each side below the pillars

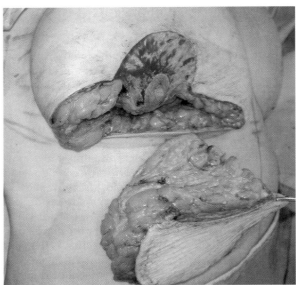

Fig. 4.15. Remaining breast tissue following resection with resected specimen lying on abdominal wall below breast

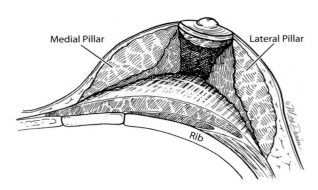

Fig. 4.16. Medial and lateral pillars viewed from below

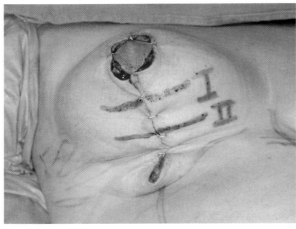

Fig. 4.17. Temporary closure – the skin is brought together with staples, and hash marks are made and numbered to facilitate definitive closure

longer the superior pedicle, the thinner it should be. The entire volume of breast tissue to be resected is then removed in one block (Fig. 4.15).

I do not use liposuction to reduce the size of the breast. The liposuction is performed toward the end of the procedure on the lateral chest wall only. Occasionally, and with a long superior pedicle, liposuction may be useful to facilitate nipple-areola inset. At this stage of the operation, I will bring the medial and lateral pillars together with my hand and assess the volume of remaining breast tissue as well as shape and projection (Fig. 4.16). If liposuction of the lateral chest wall and axillary tail is required, at this stage we will infiltrate those areas with a wetting solution. The solution consists of Ringer's lactate and to each liter is

added 250 mg xylocaine and 1 mg epinephrine. The liposuction is performed after the medial and lateral pillars are approximated.

At this stage, the nipple is brought up into the new areola and stapled in place, and the skin is temporarily closed with staples. The operation is repeated in a similar fashion on the opposite side, and then the patient is placed in a sitting position. If the volume and skin resection are adequate, then the skin margins are marked and a cross hatch is placed at two different levels to facilitate final closure (Fig. 4.17). If more breast tissue is to be resected or if the skin is redundant and more skin excision is required, the markings are made, the patient is placed recumbent, and the skin resection and/or breast resection is performed as needed. The pectoralis muscle and breast tissue are infiltrated with

10 ml marcaine 1/4% with epinephrine for postoperative anesthesia and comfort (Fig. 4.18).

Closure

Once I am satisfied that the resection has been adequate and the two breasts are closely symmetrical in shape, size, and projection, the definitive closure is performed. The medial and lateral pillars are brought together according to the cross hatch markings using 2–0 vicryl sutures. Several sutures are used to bring these pillars together. I feel this is a vital step in this procedure as it not only defines the shape and projection of the breast, but it also, I believe, contributes to the longevity of the result (Figs. 4.19, 4.20).

A small 7-mm drain is then introduced and placed between the pillars, and the tubing is exteriorized. The drain will stay in for up to 24 h. If needed, at this stage liposuction is performed (Fig. 4.21). Then the nipple and areola are inset and sutured in two layers with buried 5–0 Monocryl sutures and intracuticular 5–0 Monocryl sutures. The vertical incision is closed with 3–0 Monocryl and intracuticular 3–0 Monocryl in two layers.

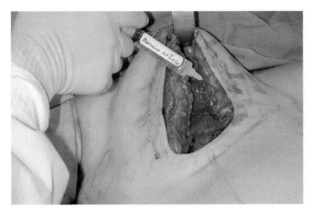

Fig. 4.18. Prior to definitive closure the pectoralis muscle and breast tissue are infiltrated with 10 ml marcaine 1/4% with epinephrine

Fig. 4.19 a-c. Definitive closure. **a** The nipple is temporarily stapled in position and a suture placed through the upper border of the vertical scar. **b** The medial and lateral pillars are brought together with a 2–0 Vicryl or PDS suture. **c** The lower end is closed with a purse-string suture

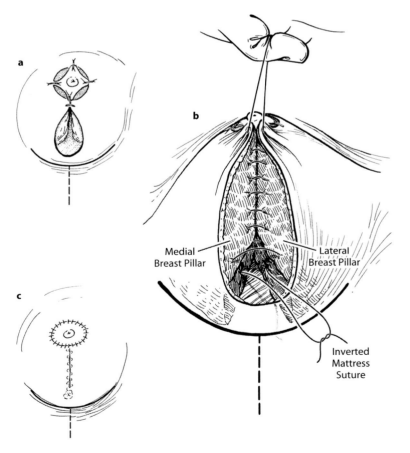

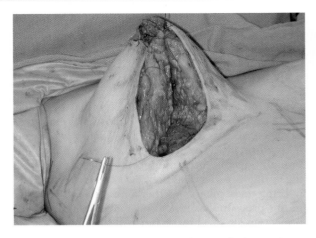

Fig. 4.20. With the initial suture holding up the breast tissue, the medial and lateral pillars are sutured together

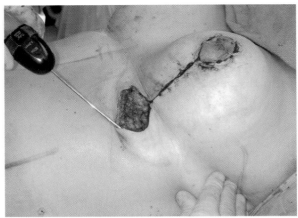

Fig. 4.21. Prior to closure of the lower end of the vertical scar liposuction of the lateral chest wall and axillary tail is performed

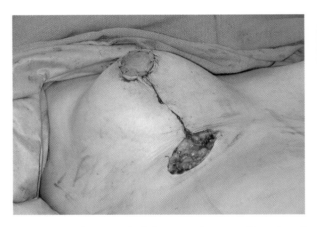

Fig. 4.22. The lower end of the vertical scar is thinned, and excess skin is excised and prepared for the purse-string suture

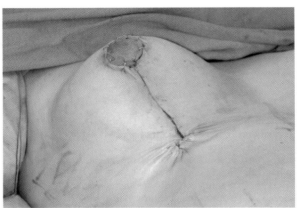

Fig. 4.23. The purse-string suture has been tied

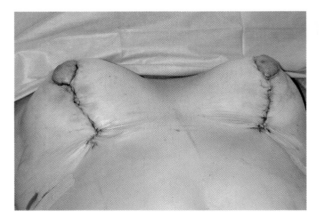

Fig. 4.24. The appearance of both breasts at the conclusion of the procedure

Management of the Lower End of the Vertical Scar

One of the most challenging components of the vertical reduction is the management of the excess skin at the lower end of the vertical scar. The choices for closure in this area include undermining the skin edges and the vertical purse string described by Lejour, the modified purse string described by Marconi and Cavina, or the short horizontal T described by Marchac.

I do not separate the skin from the underlying breast parenchyma as I believe this increases the risk of delayed wound healing, seroma, and wound disruption. I close the lower end by reducing the amount of excess skin and fat (Fig. 4.22) and then inserting a purse-string suture as described by Marconi and Cavina (Figs. 4.23, 4.24).

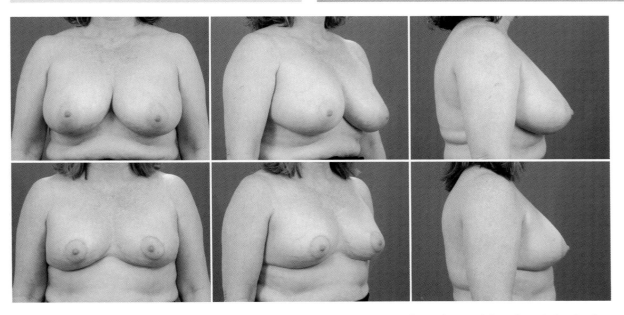

Fig. 4.25. Pre- and postoperative views, 9 months postop, of a 51-year-old woman who underwent bilateral vertical reduction. Volume of resection 432 g left breast, 388 g right breast, with 300 ml of liposuction

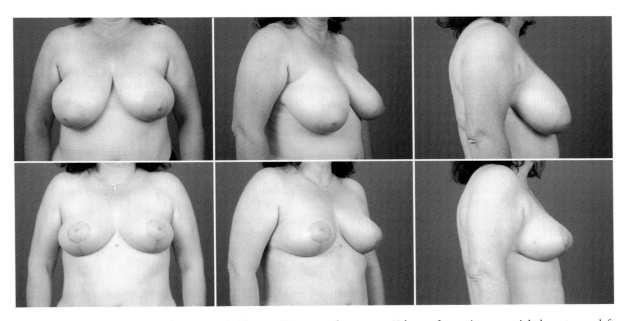

Fig. 4.26. 55-year-old woman with asymmetrical breasts. Postop result at 2 years. Volume of resection 500 g right breast, 439 g left breast, with 300 ml of liposuction

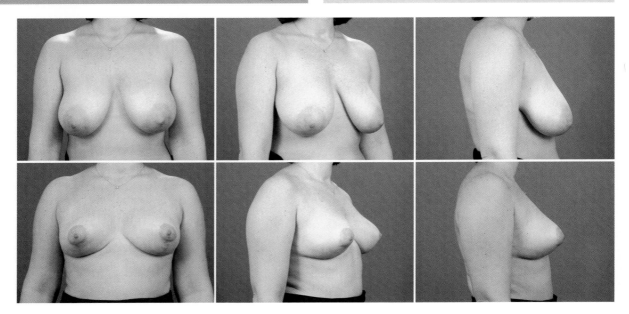

Fig. 4.27. 31-year-old woman with breast ptosis and hypertrophy, 436 g resection right breast, 478 g resection left breast, and 100 cc of liposuction. Postoperative views at 18 months. She underwent minor revision of both areola in the interim

Dressings

The suture lines are taped, and the drains are secured. The purse string at the lower end is not taped, and a piece of nonadhesive gauze is placed on it. Light dressings are applied, and the patient is put in a bra, which she will wear day and night for up to 3 weeks.

Postoperative Care

The patient is admitted overnight. The next morning the drains are removed and the patient is discharged. She is to wear the bra day and night for up to 3 weeks. The patient is advised that the breast will be full superiorly and flat below the nipple with perhaps exaggerated projection. The patient is reassured that the shape will gradually change over a few weeks. This will already have been explained to the patient during the preoperative counseling, so she will not be surprised with the immediate postoperative appearance of her breasts.

Conclusions

The vertical technique in my hands has not only reduced scar but improved shape. The breast has significantly more projection and less tendency to "bottom out" over time. It has been extremely well accepted by patients who have referred other patients for similar procedures. No operation is complication or trouble free. No operation is free of secondary revision, either! The vertical technique is no exception. I have performed revisions and had complications. These are discussed in a separate chapter.

Tips That Make a Difference

The following is a list of "tips" that in my opinion have made a big difference in improving results, minimizing complications and revisions.
- In patient selection, size is not the issue.
- Skin quantity is the issue in patient selection.
- Mark the new nipple position 2–3 cm lower than other techniques.
- Mark the upper border of the new areola at the level of the preexisting inframammary fold.
- Preserve the preexisting inframammary fold.
- Take out a triangular segment of tissue at the base of each pillar inferiorly.
- Before closure infiltrate the breast tissue and pectoralis with a dilute marcaine, 1/4% solution, for patient comfort.
- Approximate the pillars with sutures.
- Do not undermine skin flap.
- Limit liposuction to lateral chest wall.

References

1. Lassus C (1969) Possibilites et limites de la chirurgie plastique de la silhouette feminine. L'Hospital 801:575
2. Lassus C (1970) A technique for breast reduction. Int Surg 53:69
3. Lassus C (1977) New refinements in vertical mammoplasty. In: the 2nd congress of the Asian section of the International Plastic and Reconstructive Surgery Society, Tokyo
4. Lassus C (1981) New refinements in vertical mammoplasty. Chir Plast 6:81
5. Lassus C (1987) Breast reduction: evolution of a technique. A single vertical scar. Aesthetic Plast Surg 11:107
6. Lassus C (1996) A 30-year experience with vertical mammoplasty. Plast Reconstr Surg 97:373
7. Lejour M, Abboud M, Declety A, Kertesz P (1990) Reduction des cicatrices de plastie mammaire de l'ancre courte a la verticale. Ann Chir Plast Esthet 35:369
8. Lejour M (1994) Vertical mammoplasty and liposuction of the breast. Quality Medical Publishing, St Louis
9. Lejour M (1994) Vertical mammoplasty and liposuction of the breast. Plast Reconstr Surg 94:100
10. Marchac D, de Olarte G (1982) Reduction mammoplasty and correction of ptosis with a short inframammary scar. Plast Reconstr Surg 69:45
11. Marconi F, Cavina C (1993) Reduction mammoplasty and correction of ptosis: a personal technique. Plast Reconstr Surg 9:1046
12. Nahai F (1999) Vertical reduction. Operative Techniques Plast Reconstr Surg 6:97

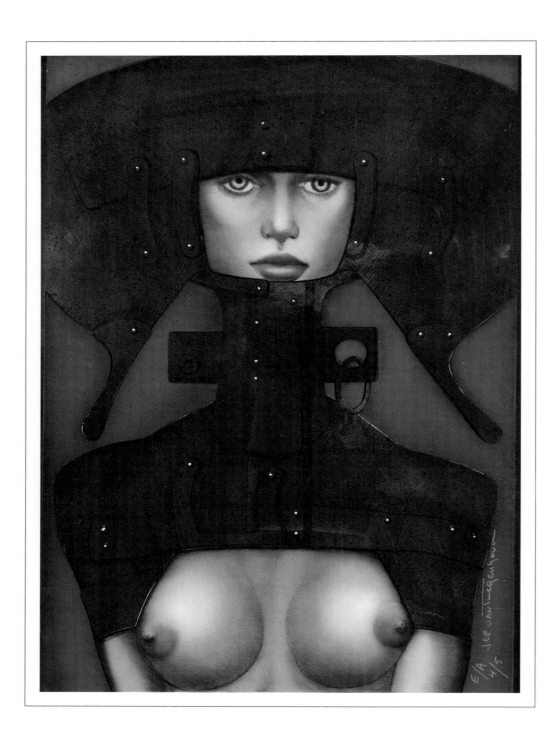

Vertical Scar Mammaplasty with a Superior Pedicle

5

Albert De Mey

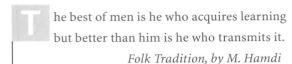

> The best of men is he who acquires learning but better than him is he who transmits it.
>
> *Folk Tradition, by M. Hamdi*

Introduction

The goal of breast reduction is the correction of the volume, shape, and symmetry of the breast while preserving nipple sensitivity. Since the early days of breast surgery, many surgical techniques have been proposed to reach this goal, but over the two last decades, new techniques have been published that attempt to minimize the scars. The periareolar scar is unavoidable as the nipple-areola complex has to be repositioned, but the vertical scar has proved to be avoidable in mastopexies [6], as has the horizontal submammary scar in the majority of cases, even in large reductions [3]. Following the description of Dartigues in 1925 and the publication of Lassus in 1970 [8], in the early 1990s Lejour popularized a technique derived from Lassus [9].

The Lejour vertical mammaplasty is a technique that combines a superior pedicle for the areola and a central resection for the breast reduction associated with liposuction and wide undermining of the skin along the vertical scar. Despite the results reported on large series [12], many surgeons are still reluctant to apply the Lejour vertical mammaplasty as a standard technique. This can be due to the use of a superior pedicle for the NAC, an inferomedial resection, and different approaches to the skin and to the glandular tissue. Moreover, the result is not obtained immediately.

The Lejour technique has been used in our department as the only technique for breast reduction since 1990. The first reports of Lejour were encouraging and confirmed by long series and late results [13]. However, at the university hospital, using the same procedure we observed up to 30 % minor complications and 15 % major complications [3]. This difference was probably due to the different populations (larger breasts, obese patients) and to the lack of experience of the surgeons in training who performed the operation in the university hospital. The same unfavorable results were published by Pickford [15]. Therefore, we tried to make the technique safer, keeping in mind the basic principles of the vertical scar mammaplasty.

Operative Technique (Figs. 5.1–5.12)

Drawings

The preoperative drawings are done the day before surgery, according to the description of Lejour [11], in a standing position. The future nipple site is positioned on a line joining the suprasternal notch with the nipple slightly lower than the inframammary fold (IMF) as projected onto the face of the breast by the index finger (Fig. 5.1).

The areolar circumference is then defined by marking the upper pole on the line drawn from the nipple to the sternal notch 2 cm above the nipple site. This distance between the sternal notch and the areolar site is 18 to 22 cm. The internal limit is positioned at 9 to 10 cm of the midline based on the width of the

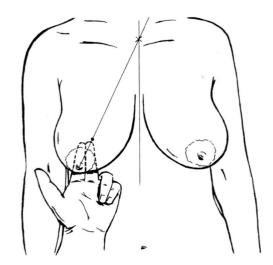

Fig. 5.1. The index finger maneuver to determine the future nipple site

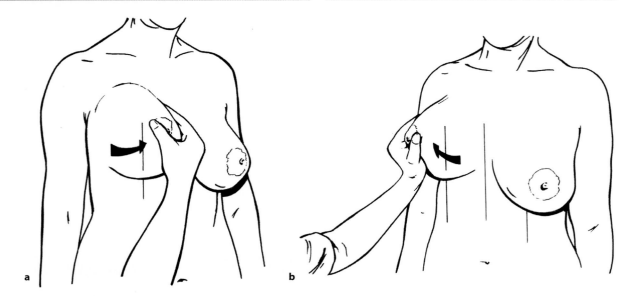

Fig. 5.2 a, b. The lateral markings are made by pushing the breast laterally and medially with an upward rotation movement

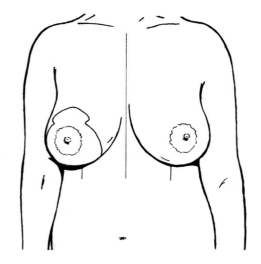

Fig. 5.3. The drawing is complete with the dome-shaped areola

chest and the external limit 7 to 8 cm externally of this point on a horizontal line drawn 3 to 4 cm below the upper marking. These three points are joined and mark the superior areolar circumference.

The inframammary fold is marked, as is the vertical axis of the breast. The lateral markings are made pushing the breast laterally and medially with an upward rotation movement, in continuity with the vertical axis drawn below the breast (Fig. 5.2a, b). The lower limits of the areola are then delineated by drawing a slightly curved line between the previous areolar points and the vertical lines. The total circumference

of the areola should measure between 14 and 16 cm to match the 4.2-cm areola template (Fig. 5.3). The same markings are made on the opposite breast. To check the symmetry of the drawings, both breasts can be gently pushed together toward the midline, making the medial markings touch.

Surgical Technique

Under general anesthesia, the patient is positioned in a semisitting position, with hands placed under the buttocks. The base of the breast is constricted with an autofixed band mammostat, and the periareolar area is deepithelialized (Fig. 5.4). Two points are then marked on each vertical line 7 to 8 cm below the lower areolar point in order to determine the height of the remaining glandular pillars (Fig. 5.5a, b). A skin hook is placed at this point and another at the lowest part of the drawings near the inframammary fold. This allows for undermining of the lower part of the breast subdermally, leaving a little adipose/glandular tissue attached to the dermis down to the inframammary fold (Fig. 5.6a, b). This dissection is performed both medially and laterally in the same position.

The dissection continues upward on the pectoralis fascia centrally, in the retromammary space, toward the subclavicular area. This dissection should not be extended laterally so as to preserve the blood supply and the innervation. A hand is then placed in the retromammary space and the breast tissue is incised vertically along the medial and lateral skin marks (Fig. 5.7). Doing this creates two glandular pillars. In a

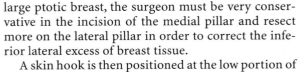

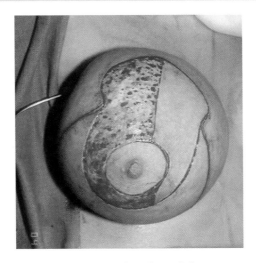

Fig. 5.4. Deepithelialization of areolar pedicle

large ptotic breast, the surgeon must be very conservative in the incision of the medial pillar and resect more on the lateral pillar in order to correct the inferior lateral excess of breast tissue.

A skin hook is then positioned at the low portion of the deepithelialized area around the areola, and the central portion of breast tissue is resected in a conical fashion (Fig. 5.8). The closure starts with a first stitch positioned at the upper pole of the areola with 4–0 nonabsorbable sutures and the second at the lower pole of the areola. Then, two last stitches are placed at 3 h and 9 h to finish the positioning of the areola (Fig. 5.9).

No sutures are placed on the pectoralis fascia except in very large fatty breasts in order to facilitate the shaping of the breast by releasing some tension. The parenchymal sutures are then inserted with heavy absorbable sutures starting at the upper part of the glan-

Fig. 5.5 a, b. 7-cm mark along vertical scar to determine dimensions of glandular pillar

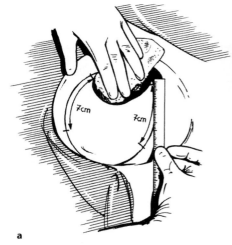

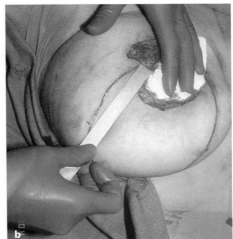

Fig. 5.6 a, b. Skin undermining of gland

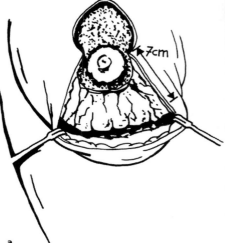

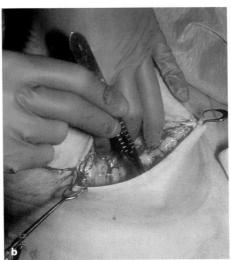

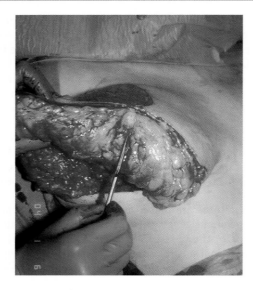

Fig. 5.7. Incision of glandular pillars

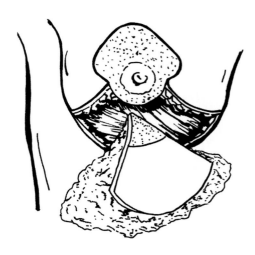

Fig. 5.8. Conical shape of central resection and lateral extensions

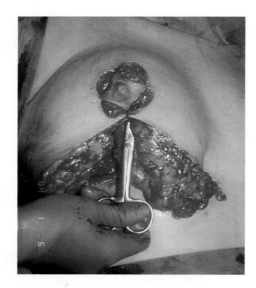

Fig. 5.9. Positioning of arc

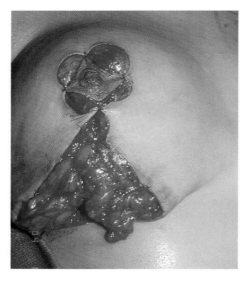

Fig. 5.10. Shaping of breast by suture of glandular pillars

dular pillars, from deep to superficial, to achieve the desired conical shape of the breast (Fig. 5.10). If necessary, some additional resection can be performed laterally and medially at the lower end of the pillars to obtain a more curved shape of the breast at the inframammary fold. Finally, a suture is placed at the lowest part of the pillars including the chest wall tissue.

A very conservative undermining of the skin is performed along the vertical scar in a triangular fashion in order to release tension on the subdermal stitches (Fig. 5.11a, b). These are done with 3.0 absorbable sutures starting at the upper end of the vertical scar as a

running suture, creating multiple fine wrinkles evenly distributed along the vertical scar. The end of this suture is attached at the base of the glandular pillars after placement of a suction drain (Fig. 5.12a, b).

There is no true contraindication for the vertical mammaplasty. However, as in any breast reduction technique, care must be taken in special occasions. The superior pedicle technique has proved reliable in large breasts. However, in elderly obese patients needing a large reduction, the Thorek amputation is probably more advisable. In large reductions, care must be taken to widen the areolar pedicle in accordance with

Fig. 5.11 a, b. Subcutaneous suture along vertical scar with even puckering of excess of skin

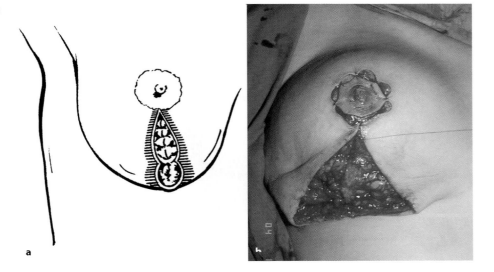

Fig. 5.12 a, b. Final aspect of breast at end of operation

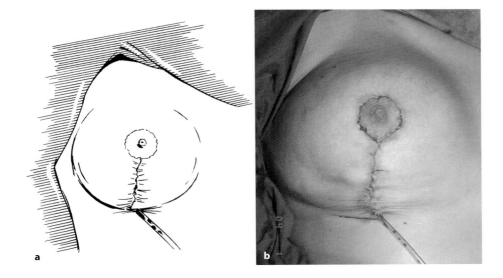

its length. This can be easily done during the preoperative drawings: after positioning the internal border of the areola, the external limit can be placed 8 to 9 cm from the first mark. This allows for a very safe 16- to 18-cm-long areolar pedicle.

In some large resections (1000 g/breast), a small horizontal skin excision is performed in the inframammary fold at the end of the vertical suture in order to avoid crossing the inframammary fold or leaving a dog ear (Fig. 5.15.). This is recommended in patients with redundant skin and limited skin elasticity or presenting risk factors such as smoking or diabetes. The skin is then sutured with 3.0 nonabsorbable stitches. A light dressing is applied on the wounds, with an additional roll of gauze placed in the lower part of the breast to avoid a dead space in the under-

mined areas. This technique differs from the original technique, as proposed by Lejour, in the absence of liposuction and of skin undermining on the glandular pillars. Moreover, skin puckering is limited and thick skin folds or dog ears are avoided at the level of the inframammary fold.

Results

From 1996 to 2002, 261 patients were operated on at the university hospital using the vertical mammaplasty as described above. The mean age was 34 years (14–68 years). The average weight resection was 530 g (0 to 3480 g) per breast, and the mean BMI was 26.6 UI (18 to 45 UI).

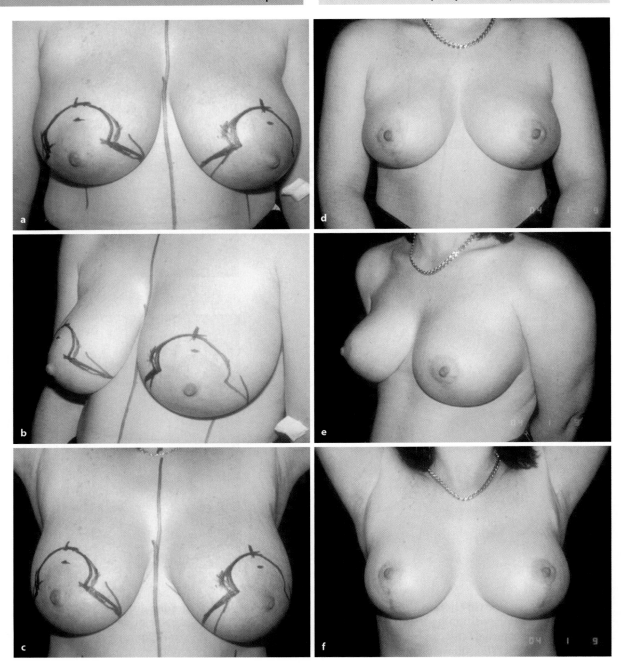

Fig. 5.13. a–c Preoperative views. **d–f** Postoperative views at 1 year after resection of 250 g on right and 300 g on left breast

Short Scar Periareolar Inferior Pedicle Reduction (SPAIR) Mammaplasty

6

DENNIS C. HAMMOND

> **B**reast reduction offers an opportunity rarely seen in plastic surgery, for not only is there too much volume, there is too much skin. With a sound operative strategy, excellent technique, and a discerning artistic eye, the sculpting of an artistic and stable breast shape can occur every time, and now we can do it with half the scar! What an exciting time to be a plastic surgeon.
>
> *Dennis Hammond*

Introduction

Any operative procedure designed to reduce the enlarged breast can be described as having four interrelated components. First, the volume of the breast must be reduced, leaving behind strategically located tissue that will create an aesthetic breast shape. Second, the excessively large skin envelope must be reduced, leaving behind enough skin to cover the reduced breast. Third, a pedicle of tissue must be created that will reliably maintain blood supply to the nipple and areola. Fourth, an aesthetic shape must be created, either passively or with some sort of shaping maneuver. The most common procedure for breast reduction satisfies these requirements by basing the blood supply to the nipple and areola on an inferior pedicle, resecting parenchyma peripherally around the pedicle, using an inverted T-type of skin pattern to manage the excess skin envelope, and passively shaping the breast by closing the flaps around the inferior pedicle and allowing postoperative settling to "shape" the breast. This procedure, also referred to as the "Wise" pattern inferior pedicle breast reduction, has stood the test of time as a reliable and versatile method of breast reduction.

However, with the description of various reduced scar techniques of breast reduction [1–11], the well-documented complications associated with the Wise pattern technique have been thrown into sharper focus. Specifically, the inframammary scar can be problematic in some patients, with the medial and lateral portions of the scar being prone to hypertrophy. Additionally, the postoperative shape change associated with the Wise pattern technique can occasionally spill over from simple postoperative settling into a shape distortion known as "bottoming out." Taken together, these two complications can adversely affect the overall result after breast reduction.

Recent advances in breast reduction technique have attempted to address these problems by reducing the amount of cutaneous scar while preserving aesthetic breast shape. The focus of this chapter will be to describe a reduced scar technique based on an inferior pedicle called the short scar periareolar inferior pedicle reduction (SPAIR) mammaplasty.

Operative Strategy

The SPAIR mammaplasty bases the blood supply to the nipple and areola on an inferior pedicle with parenchyma being removed from around the periphery of the pedicle in the shape of a horseshoe. Skin is resected in a circumvertical pattern that limits the scar to the central portion of the breast and avoids the more traditional long inframammary scar. By reducing the circumference of the periareolar incision with the vertical skin component, large periareolar patterns can be managed without excessive pleating or distortion of the periareolar closure. In addition, the vertical component tends to produce a coning effect, which enhances the overall shape of the breast. Shaping is accomplished with internal suturing of both the flaps and the pedicle. By combining these surgical maneuvers, a wide variety of breast problems ranging from simple ptosis to severe macromastia can be effectively and reliably managed [12–15].

Marking

The goal of the marking procedure is to accurately identify the appropriate amount of skin to leave behind that will effectively wrap around the inferior pedicle and assist in shaping the breast. To organize

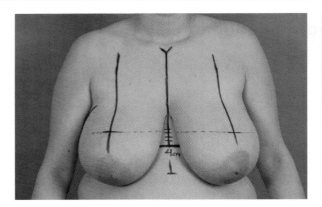

Fig. 6.1. The inframammary fold location is identified with a line connecting the folds across the midline. Measuring up 4 cm from this mark, a horizontal line is drawn and, where this line intersects the breast meridian, identifies the top of the periareolar pattern

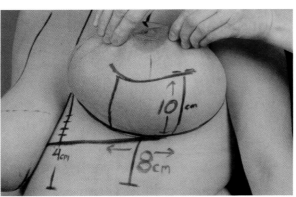

Fig. 6.2. An 8-cm pedicle is centered on the breast meridian. On either side of the pedicle, a distance of 8 to 10 cm is measured up from the fold, and these two points are communicated in a line that parallels the inframammary fold. This creates a rectangular-shaped segment of skin that defines the limits of the inferior skin envelope

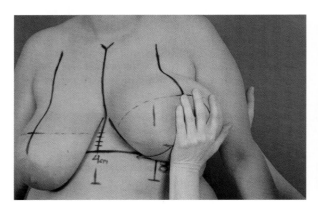

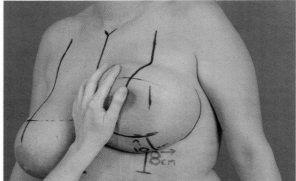

Figs. 6.3, 6.4. By drawing the breast first up and out, and then up and in, the breast meridian can be transposed onto the breast at the level of the nipple to identify the medial and lateral points of the pattern

this process, the breast is divided into four sections. With the patient upright, the sternal midline, the inframammary fold, and the lateral margin of the breast are marked. The inframammary fold mark is communicated across the midline so that with the breasts in repose the exact location of the fold can be seen without any distortion caused by lifting or otherwise manipulating the breast. The breast meridian is visualized and marked as it defines the longitudinal axis of the breast. This line extends from the clavicle down to and below the inframammary fold. The top of the periareolar pattern is marked by measuring up from the inframammary fold 4 cm in the midline. A horizontal line is drawn across the chest at this point and, where this line intersects the breast meridian, identifies the top of the pattern (Fig. 6.1). This point can be checked

by using the familiar maneuver of placing the fingers of the left hand under the breast and palpating with the fingers of the right hand anteriorly on the breast to estimate the location of the fold. Alternatively, a direct measurement from the midpoint of the clavicle down to this uppermost mark can be made, with this distance measuring 21–24 cm in most patients.

The inferior skin envelope is determined by direct measurement. An 8-cm pedicle width is diagrammed centered on the breast meridian. On either side of the pedicle and extending from the inframammary fold upward, a measurement of 8 to 10 cm is made. These two marks are then smoothly communicated in a line that parallels the inframammary fold (Fig. 6.2). This identifies the skin envelope that will be maintained inferiorly, with the 8-cm longitudinal measurement being

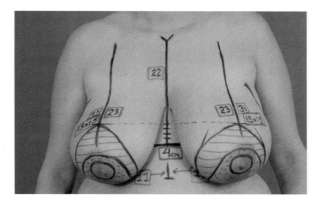

Fig. 6.5. The final marking pattern with the skin to be resected (*crosshatched*) and the skin of the inferior pedicle to be deepithelialized (*dotted*)

used in cases of mastopexy and small reductions of less than 400 g and the 10-cm measurement being used in reductions of 800 g or more.

The medial and lateral portions of the periareolar pattern are determined by gently lifting the breast with the left hand up and out, and then up and in, thus allowing the breast meridian to be transposed onto the medial and lateral breast skin level with the nipple (Figs. 6.3, 6.4). This maneuver is designed to mimic what the breast will look like once it is reduced, so when lifting the breast slight pressure is applied to create a rounded contour laterally and medially before marking the lateral and medial portions of the periareolar pattern. Marking these points in this fashion ensures that enough skin will be preserved medially and laterally to comfortably wrap around the inferior pedicle after reduction without creating undue tension. A measurement can be made from the midsternal line to the medial mark at the level of the nipple, and this distance should measure at least 12 cm in most cases.

Once these four landmarks are identified, they are smoothly joined together to create an elongated oval. The inferior pedicle is drawn in with the superior portion of the pedicle skirting the areola by a distance of 2 cm. It is helpful conceptually to crosshatch the skin that will be removed from around the pedicle and identify the skin of the inferior pedicle to be deepithelialized with dots (Fig. 6.5). A final measurement is made reflecting the width and length of the periareolar pattern. This measurement is helpful as a guide in predicting the difficulty of managing the redundant skin envelope of the breast. Measurements of 15 cm or less pose little difficulty in breast shaping, while measurements of 15 to 20 cm can occasionally cause difficulty. In cases where the dimensions of the periareolar pattern measure more than 20 cm, experience with the technique is required to obtain the optimal result.

Operative Technique

Generally speaking, most cases of breast reduction in my practice are still performed under general anesthesia and include an overnight stay in the hospital. However, cases of mastopexy and smaller reductions of 500 g or less are often performed in an outpatient setting. In preparing for the SPAIR procedure, several details are best managed ahead of time. Inherent in the SPAIR procedure is assessment of the shape of the breast during the procedure, as one of the operative goals is to create an aesthetically appealing breast immediately. This must be done with the patient upright at least 80°. Therefore, an operative table that will sit up to this degree is mandatory.

Preoperative communication with the anesthesiologist will facilitate fluid management of the patient to allow the sitting position without creating significant hypotension. A long ventilatory circuit will also allow the upright positioning of the patient to be accomplished without excessive manipulation by the anesthesiologist. The arms of the patient are extended outward 90° on padded arm boards and are gently secured with towels and gauze wraps. The head is supported on a foam headrest, and the knees are supported by a pillow to ease strain on the back. During the draping of the chest, care is taken to ensure that the tops of the shoulders can be seen to make certain that malposition of the shoulders does not adversely influence the correct assessment of nipple-areola complex position or the location of the inframammary fold.

The procedure is begun by injecting the margins of the proposed incisions and the areas to be initially deepithelialized with a diluted solution of lidocaine with epinephrine. This dramatically reduces oozing, particularly in the area of the inferior pedicle. A breast tourniquet is applied and the center of the nipple marked. Using a multidiameter areola marker, a circle measuring 52 mm in diameter is marked on the existing areola. Most patients undergoing breast reduction can accommodate this measurement with the areola under stretch without difficulty. When the areola is smaller than 52 mm, the initial incision is made as big as the existing areola allows. The strategy behind this measurement is to make the initial areolar incision larger than the ultimate periareolar defect. Since the diameter of the periareolar defect will be controlled with the Gore-Tex purse-string suture, and this defect will be sized at 40–44 mm, little tension will be applied to the areola, thus allowing the 52-mm areola to rest comfortably within the 44-mm opening. This avoids a stretched-out or pasted-on appearance to the nipple-areola complex.

Initial incisions around the areola, inferior pedicle, and periareolar pattern are now made. The inferior

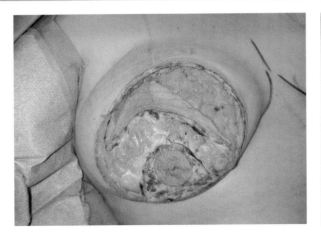

Fig. 6.6. Appearance of the breast after deepithelialization of the inferior pedicle and medial, superior, and lateral flap creation

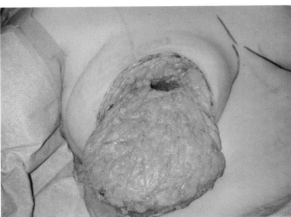

Fig. 6.7. After the flaps have been developed, the excess breast tissue, along with the inferior pedicle, can be essentially delivered from within the confines of the flaps. The flaps themselves have volume and structure that contribute to the overall shape of the breast

pedicle within the periareolar pattern is deepithelialized, as is a 5-mm segment of skin around the periphery of the periareolar pattern. Bovie cautery is used from this point on to complete the remainder of the procedure. The dermis is divided around the inferior pedicle and around the periphery of the periareolar pattern at a point 5 mm in and away from the initial epidermal incision. This creates a 5-mm dermal shelf into which the Gore-Tex purse-string suture will eventually be placed. The tourniquet is released and the medial, superior, and lateral flaps are developed.

Initial flap dissection is performed directly under the dermis around the periareolar pattern from the lateral border of the pedicle around to the medial border. It is here that most bleeding will be encountered as there are often large veins coursing radially away from the center of the breast. After the dermal shelf has been developed, dissection gradually angles down to the chest wall medially and superiorly until the pectoralis major fascia is identified. The thickness of the flaps at the base of the breast medially and superiorly is generally 4 to 6 cm. Laterally, dissection is performed at the level of the breast fascia extending down to the previously marked lateral border of the breast. In this manner, a flap 2 to 3 cm thick is created, with the dissection merging smoothly with the thicker superior flap. Care is taken to be certain that flap dissection extends down to the medial and lateral base of the inferior pedicle, without inadvertent undermining of the pedicle (Fig. 6.6).

The end result of this dissection strategy is the creation of a thin initial flap that will wrap around the inferior pedicle without tension or tissue crowding around the areola. As the flaps become thicker, the su-

perior and medial borders of the breast become defined and, along with the inferior pedicle, significantly determine the overall shape of the breast. Experience has shown that if the lateral flap is kept too thick, excessive lateral fullness will result, creating an overly wide, "boxy" appearance to the breast. At this point the bulk of the breast has been essentially delivered from within the confines of the flaps (Fig. 6.7). The inferior pedicle is now skeletonized, evenly removing the redundant tissue from around the nipple and areola. Again, care is taken not to undermine the pedicle. This is the same maneuver that is performed in the traditional inferior pedicle Wise pattern breast reduction.

After removal, the specimen has the shape of an elongated horseshoe that is slightly longer laterally than medially. Once the breast has been reduced, the remaining parenchyma is prepared for the placement of shaping sutures. The upper flap is undermined at the level of the pectoralis major fascia for a distance of 6 to 8 cm. Likewise, the medial flap is undermined up to but not past the internal mammary perforators. The ledge created along the upper flap junction with the pectoralis major, where undermining was initiated, is then transposed superiorly and sutured to the pectoralis fascia. This has the effect of using the patient's own breast parenchyma to autoaugment the upper pole of the breast and correct any preoperative upper pole concavity. Often only one suture of 3–0 monofilament is required, although as many as three sutures may be required in cases of extreme ptosis to adequately fill in the upper pole of the breast. It is sometimes helpful to perform this shaping maneuver with the patient upright

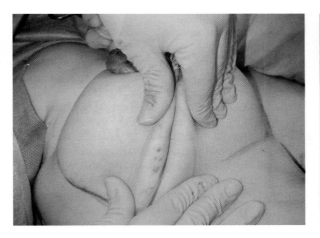

Fig. 6.8. After removal of breast tissue from around the pedicle, the redundant inferior pole skin is plicated upon itself to create a smooth rounded inferior pole contour

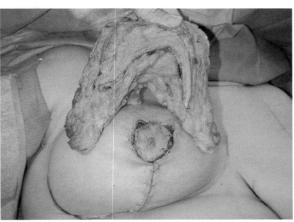

Fig. 6.9. With removal of excess tissue from around the inferior pedicle, the resected specimen is seen to have the shape of a horseshoe. In addition, the inferior pole of the breast has been plicated together to create a smooth, even contour

so the immediate effect of the flap transposition can be seen.

Next, the same ledge medially is plicated to itself with one suture. This has the effect of gathering the base of the medial flap to help create a rounded appearance in the breast medially. Lastly, the base of the inferior pedicle is sutured centrally to the pectoralis fascia. This helps centralize the pedicle and keeps it from tending to fall off laterally, resulting in loss of projection and excess lateral fullness. Breast reshaping with these sutures is performed only in cases of excess concavity in the upper pole of the breast preoperatively. Some patients, particularly those who are over their ideal body weight by 20 pounds or more, actually present with no upper pole concavity and therefore do not require the extra flap mobilization as described. In these cases, the inferior pedicle is simply sutured into position centrally and the operation proceeds.

The patient is now brought into a sitting position of 60°, and the upper portion of the pedicle is grasped with a heavy clamp. Traction is exerted upwards on the pedicle until the tissues on either side of the pedicle begin to fold. Two small folds in the skin envelope are created by this maneuver, and the inferior margins of these folds are grasped and stapled together. This point is called the key staple point as it sets the remainder of the inferior skin pattern. A hemostat is applied to the deepithelialized dermal border next to the staple, and again upward traction is now applied to the skin envelope of the lower pole of the breast. The redundant skin is plicated together progressively, again with staples, until a smooth, even, and aesthetic breast contour is created (Figs. 6.8, 6.9). The medial

skin margin will be longer than the lateral skin margin, which necessitates making a gradual adjustment as these staples are placed. It is best to take up the major portion of the length discrepancy in the central portion of the vertical plication as it makes the overall shaping of the inferior pole easier.

An attempt is made to not extend the plication line below the inframammary fold. If further skin plication is required, as often happens in reductions larger than 500 g, then the plication is gently curved out laterally until the desired shape is created. Only in cases of mastopexy or reductions of less than 400 g does the vertical incision run straight down to the inframammary fold as in the classical vertical mammaplasty. Once an acceptable shape has been created, the skin plication line is marked with a surgical marker and cross hatches are marked to aid in closing the inferior incision. The staples are removed, revealing a wedge-shaped segment of the inferior skin envelope that will need to be removed in order to remove the redundant skin and cone the breast. In the region of the inferior pedicle, the skin is simply deepithelialized. Medial and lateral to the inferior pedicle, a full-thickness wedge of skin and parenchyma is removed. Typically this involves only a small segment of tissue medially, but laterally the entire length of the inferior skin flap is eventually incised. This full-thickness release of the lateral flap facilitates subsequent transposition of the lateral flap on top of the deepithelialized inferior pedicle as it is joined to the medial flap during closure of the vertical segment, thus preventing bunching or gathering of tissue during closure, which can distort the shape of the lower pole of the breast. If desired, a drain is placed at this point and brought out through an inferolateral stab incision. Drains are typically used in reductions of 800 g or more. The vertical incision is plicated back together with temporary staples and closed with 4–0 absorbable monofilament sutures placed in an inverted interrupted fashion followed by a 4–0 running subcuticular suture.

The periareolar opening is larger than the areolar diameter at this point. It is closed down with a purse-string suture of CV-3 Gore-Tex. This suture is ideally suited for this purpose as it is supple, strong, and has an extremely smooth surface, which allows it to glide easily through tissue without catching. The suture is available on a straight needle specifically designed for use as a purse-string suture. The goal of placing the suture is to use the straight needle to pass the suture directly in the substance of the dermal shelf created during flap elevation. The knot is always placed at the medial border of the periareolar opening, which allows easy identification and removal if desired at a later date. The knot must be buried below the flap; thus the suture placement is begun by passing the needle from deep to superficial and then from superficial to deep to finish. Once the purse string is completed, the suture can easily be slid around the entire periareolar opening to evenly distribute any wrinkles or pleats that may have formed to minimize their effect on the closure and maximize the likelihood that they will settle completely.

The periareolar opening is cinched down to what is usually an oval shape 35 to 40 mm in diameter. The patient is then raised into the upright position of at least 80°, and the periareolar opening will form an elongated oval extending from superomedial to inferolateral, especially in the larger reductions. This opening must be converted into more of a circular configuration. The areolar marker can be used to outline a 44-mm-diameter opening, or, alternatively, the circular diagram can be drawn freehand. The additional skin is deepithelialized, with care being taken not to inadvertently cut the Gore-Tex suture. The areola is inset into the periareolar defect with eight evenly spaced inverted interrupted 4–0 absorbable monofilament sutures followed by a running subcuticular suture around the areolar closure to finish the procedure.

Usually one breast is completed before work on the opposite breast is started; however, performing the operative steps alternatively on each breast may provide better control and enhance the likelihood of obtaining better overall symmetry, especially if any degree of preoperative asymmetry is noted. Once closure is completed, the skin edges are treated with a topical adhesive followed by wound edge support with steristrips. The incisions are dressed with clear plastic sheeting, and a support garment is applied simply for comfort and to control swelling.

Postoperative Care

A support garment is worn continuously for the first week to provide support and comfort. Drains are emptied three times a day and as needed. There is no need to change dressings as the opsite dressing is occlusive; therefore, the patient can shower the day after surgery. At 7 to 10 days postoperatively, the patient is seen in the office, where dressings and steristrips are removed, exposed suture ends are clipped, and drains are removed. Scar treatment begins at this visit with a vitamin E-based topical ointment covered with paper tape or silicone gel sheeting. The ointment is reapplied every 3 days and continued for 6 weeks. The patient is seen again at 6 weeks, 6 months, and 1 year to document the progress of the result. Initially the breast will have a slightly coned appearance, but the overall shape of the breast will be good. As the swelling resolves over the next 6 weeks, the breast settles into the final shape with resolution of any upper pole fullness and a pleasing rounding out of the lower pole.

It is important to note that, while swelling does subside and the breast settles over time, bottoming out in the traditional sense does not occur. Because the attachments of the inframammary fold are left intact during the procedure, there is no opening up of the loose subscarpal layer along the inframammary fold; thus the compliant fat and parenchyma of the breast cannot descend into this space, creating over time a new inframammary fold that is lower than the initial inframammary fold incision. As a result, there is no need to artificially place the nipple and areola complex in a low position to accommodate for expected "bottoming out," as is done with the Wise pattern procedure.

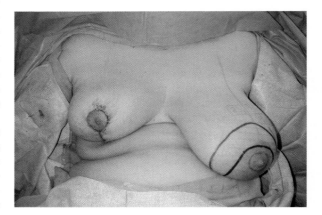

Fig. 6.10. Final appearance of the right breast after SPAIR mammaplasty. The breast base diameter has been reduced, the nipple-areola complex raised, and the upper pole fullness restored, and a pleasing contour is evident with no inferior pole notching

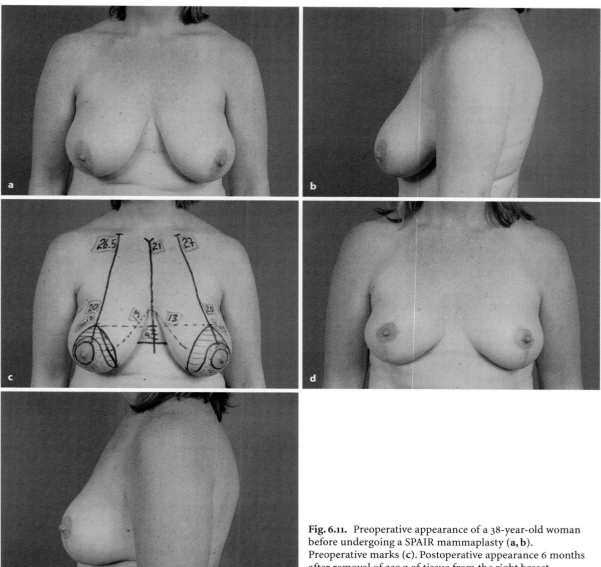

Fig. 6.11. Preoperative appearance of a 38-year-old woman before undergoing a SPAIR mammaplasty (**a, b**). Preoperative marks (**c**). Postoperative appearance 6 months after removal of 239 g of tissue from the right breast and 291 g from the left (**d, e**)

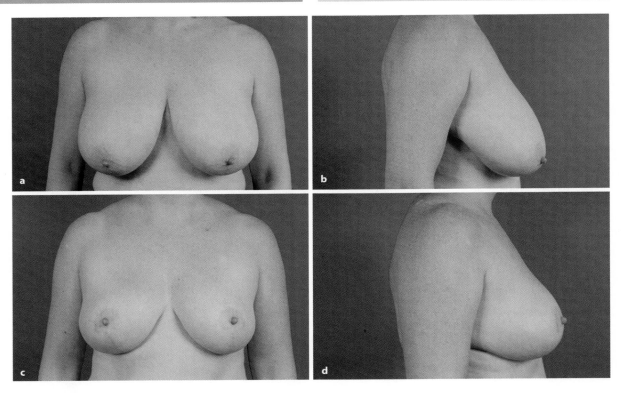

Fig. 6.12. Preoperative appearance of a 36-year-old woman before undergoing a SPAIR mammaplasty (**a, b**). Postoperative appearance 7 months after removal of 560 g of tissue from the right breast and 649 g from the left (**c, d**)

Results

The results obtained using the SPAIR mammaplasty have been uniformly satisfying to both patient and surgeon alike. Because the operative steps are essentially the same in all patients ranging from mastopexy to large reductions of 1000 g or more, the technique is easily learned and applied. The pleasing shape that is created immediately only improves with time as the breast settles and swelling resolves, a process that is usually complete by 6 months postoperatively. In most instances, this results in a slight ptosis, which accentuates what is already a very aesthetic breast shape. Scars are usually fully mature at 6 months to 1 year postoperative. Only rarely is any deleterious shape change noticed in breasts treated with this technique. Because the inframammary fold is not violated during the procedure, it does not move during the postoperative recovery period. However, in larger patients with more elastic skin, excessive stretch of the skin of the inferior pole over the stable inframammary fold is sometimes noted. This can expand the volume of the lower pole, creating pseudoptosis. This condition is easily treated with a secondary skin excision of the vertical segment once the shape has stabilized. Several patients have become pregnant after undergoing a SPAIR reduction

without experiencing a significant change in the shape of their breasts. None of these patients had any desire to breastfeed, although the ability to breastfeed should be preserved due to the use of the inferior pedicle, which remains in continuity with the nipple.

For cases of mastopexy and small reductions of less than 500 g, the technique is easily applied and the redraping of the inferior skin envelope is not difficult. The ability to reshape the breast with the internal flap sutures is a major advantage in these patients, who often have high aesthetic expectations. Being able to accomplish this reshaping with a limited scar makes the procedure appealing to many patients who are reluctant to undergo a more traditional Wise pattern procedure. For reductions of 500 to 1000 g, the inferior skin redraping requires more finesse but is usually easily accomplished. Patients with an excessive skin envelope for a given breast volume tend to be more problematic in this regard and may require more attention intraoperatively to create the desired breast shape. For reductions of more than 1000 g, it is helpful to have experience with the technique in order to achieve optimal results. For these larger patients, appropriate parenchymal resection, optimal lower pole skin redraping, and avoidance of excessive periareolar wrinkling all require operative skill to be optimally managed.

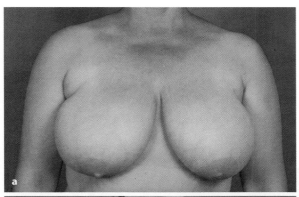

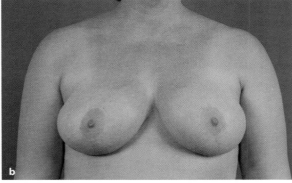

Fig. 6.13. Preoperative appearance of a 43-year-old woman before undergoing a SPAIR mammaplasty (**a**). Postoperative appearance 5 years after removal of 628 g of tissue from the right breast and 561 g from the left (**b**)

Complications

The vast majority of patients undergoing SPAIR mammaplasty heal promptly, have an aesthetic breast shape, and are happy with the results. When a complication is noted, it is most often a minor wound separation that heals secondarily over time. Fat necrosis can occur at the distal end of the inferior pedicle in larger patients and usually manifests as a periareolar mass noted 3 to 6 weeks postoperatively. The avascular fat is allowed to mature into a well-circumscribed mass over the next 6 months to 1 year and is then removed to ease subsequent cancer surveillance over time. Shape distortion is uncommon and, when noted, easily treated by removing additional skin in either the vertical or periareolar dimensions. Scar revisions are likewise possible once scarring has matured at 1 year. Persistent periareolar wrinkling can be similarly improved with a periareolar scar revision, excision of the wrinkled skin, and reclosure as before, often without the need for the Gore-Tex suture. In rare cases, the Gore-Tex suture can be the focus of a foreign body reaction or even a cellulitis. In these instances,

the suture is simply removed and the symptoms resolve. In most instances, the areola does not spread if sufficient time has passed to allow the scar to stabilize the periareolar opening, usually at least 6 weeks.

Summary

The SPAIR mammaplasty is an easily applied and technically straightforward technique for breast reduction and mastopexy that affords the advantages of aesthetic shape, reduced scar burden, and stability over time. The immediate effect of reduction and reshaping can be seen at the time of surgery with no postoperative settling period being required to assess the results of the operation. This affords the surgeon improved control over the final result. It is recommended as a consistent and reliable technique for breast reduction and mastopexy.

References

1. Lassus C (1970) A new technique for breast reduction. Int Surg 53:69
2. Lassus C (1986) An "all season" mammaplasty. Aesthetic Plast Surg 10:9
3. Lassus C (1987) Breast reduction: evolution of a technique – a single vertical scar. Aesthetic Plast Surg 11:107
4. Lassus C (1996) A 30-year experience with vertical mammaplasty. Plast Reconstr Surg 97:373
5. Lejour M, Abbound M (1990) Vertical mammaplasty without inframammary scar with breast liposuction. Perspect Plast Surg 4:67
6. Lejour M (1994) Vertical mammaplasty and liposuction of the breast. Plast Reconstr Surg 94:100
7. Peixoto G (1984) Reduction mammaplasty. Aesthetic Plast Surg 8:231
8. Arie G (1957) Una nueva tecnica de mastoplastia. Rev Latinoam Cir Plast 3:23
9. Regnault P (1974) Reduction mammaplasty by the B technique. Plast Reconstr Surg 53:19
10. Regnault P (1980) Breast reduction: B technique. Plast Reconstr Surg 65:840
11. Regnault P (1990) Breast reduction and mastopexy, an old love story: B technique update. Aesthetic Plast Surg 14:101
12. Hammond DC (1999) Short scar periareolar inferior pedicle reduction (SPAIR) mammaplasty. Plast Reconstr Surg 103:890
13. Hammond DC (1999) Short-scar periareolar-inferior pedicle reduction (SPAIR) mammaplasty: operative techniques. Plast Reconstruc Surg 6:106
14. Hammond DC (2001) Short scar periareolar inferior pedicle reduction (SPAIR) mammaplasty/mastopexy: how I do it step by step. Perspect Plast Surg 15:61
15. Hammond DC (2002) The SPAIR mammaplasty. Clin Plast Surg 29:411

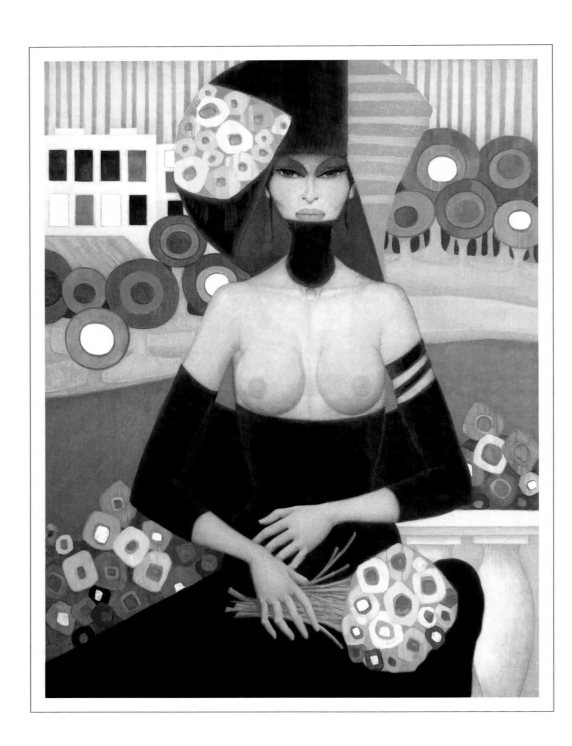

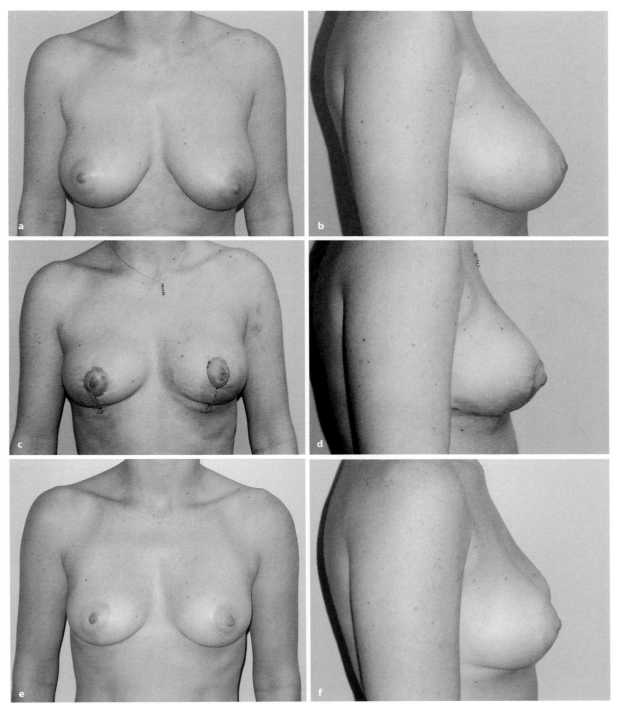

Fig. 7.10. Patient had 295 g removed from the right breast and 350 g removed from the left breast. **a** Preop frontal view. **b** Preop lateral view. **c** 10 days postop frontal view. **d** 10 days postop lateral view. **e** 18 months postop frontal view. **f** 18 months postop lateral view

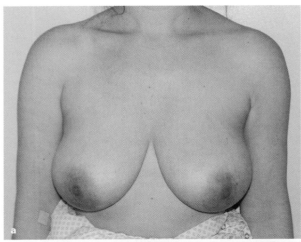

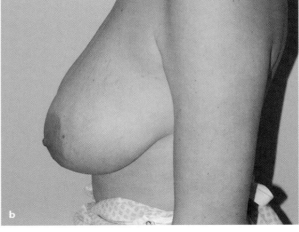

Fig. 7.11 a–g. Patient had 370 g removed from the right breast and 410 g from the left breast. **a** Preop frontal view. **b** Preop lateral view. **c** Intraoperative view at end of operation. **d** 3 weeks postop frontal view. **e** 3 weeks postop lateral view. **f** 2.5 years postop frontal view. **g** 2.5 years postop lateral view

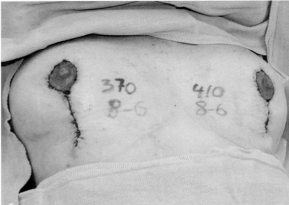

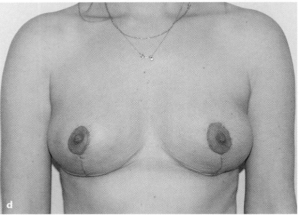

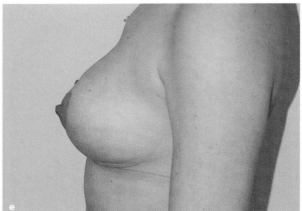

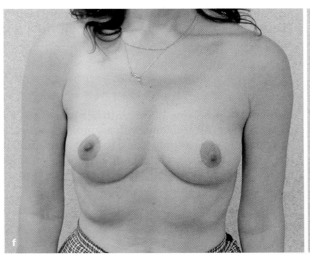
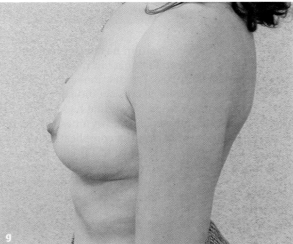

had an infection rate of about 5%. I now put all my patients on one intraoperative dose of a cephalosporin and 5 days of oral cephalexin postoperatively. Not only did my infection rate fall to less than 1%, but patients stopped calling with wound-healing problems.

Taping

I use either steristrips or, more recently, paper tape (Micropore) to cover the incisions. Because I would rather leave some gaps in the closure with my subcuticular suturing so that the skin closure is not constricted, I use the tape to approximate any final openings in the skin edges. Some surgeons tape the inferior portion of the breast to encourage the dog ear to settle. I have avoided this because of fear of causing blistering in the skin from the tape. As long as the tape is applied without tension, this may very well help the area settle faster.

Bandages and Compression

I cover the incisions with gauze only to absorb any drainage of blood through the incisions. I use a "compression" brassiere that does not really compress anything. The main reason for using a brassiere is to hold the bandages in place. I allow the patient to shower the next day – and leave the tape on for three weeks. They are then encouraged to use pantiliners in the bra for any persistent oozing. After the first 2 weeks, they can switch to a sports-type bra – preferably with a band that comes down onto the chest wall. A lycra camisole top is a good option before they feel comfortable enough to use a standard type of brassiere.

Recovery

Activities

I do not restrict patients' activities or their arm movements. They are told to let their discomfort be their guide. Patients can return to work after about 2 weeks for a desk job to about 4 weeks for anything that involves heavy lifting.

Follow-up

Because the sutures are all absorbable, the follow-up routine varies. I usually try to see the patients sometime during the first month, then at 2 or 3 months, then about 6 months, and then at 1 year. But getting patients to return for follow-up is a difficult task.

We take photographs every time we see the patient. That way, the patient can see how the shape and the puckering are settling down. All patients have been warned that any revisions must wait a full year – that almost all patients worry about the puckering, but that it needs to be corrected in less than 5% of patients.

Complications

Puckering

The most common complication is puckering. There is no question that my revision rate for the vertical approach is higher than it was for the inverted T approach. However, I am also more demanding about the result than I used to be.

Necrosis

My most serious complication has been nipple-areolar necrosis. I had been fortunate in my series of 400 inferior pedicle, inverted T reductions never to have had a full nipple-areolar necrosis. I did have one partial and some marginal problems that had healed well without intervention. As Dr. Goldwyn has repeatedly warned us, however, having the complication of nipple necrosis is just a matter of time. Initially my problems were with the superior pedicle and trying to leave it too thick. I have, however, had problems with the medial pedicle with a necrosis rate of 0.5 % of patients. Although this is comparable to published studies, it is still very difficult for both patient and surgeon.

Infection

See discussion on antibiotics in Operative Technique.

Hematoma/Seroma

One note of caution is that the tumescent type of infiltration can lead to a false sense of security. It is important to identify the leash to what would have been an inferior pedicle and to make sure that the vessels are cauterized. I have had only two patients (out of 1100) require a return to the operating room to drain a hematoma, and both resulted from delayed bleeding from these vessels. I have had only one patient in whom I had to aspirate an infected seroma and a very few others where a seroma drained spontaneously. I suspect that there are more seromas, but I don't aspirate them – they seem to settle without intervention.

Underresection/Pseudoptosis

This is the second most common reason for revision. I still have problems with underresection with this technique. I cannot get breasts as small with the vertical approach as I could with the inverted T, inferior pedicle approach. The technique itself does not allow as much resection, but the result at the end of the procedure can be misleading. The breast looks smaller than it is. If the plan is to remove about 700 g, then it is important to get as close to 700 g as possible. I will use liposuction to help get the breasts smaller, but patients still find that they were hoping for a smaller breast. A secondary procedure can often be performed with liposuction only, but a further vertical resection (breast tissue, not much skin) will help improve any pseudoptosis that remains. I firmly believe that much of the pseudoptosis that results with this approach is due underresection, not the design.

Asymmetry

Asymmetry problems occur with all breast reductions. Most of my problems with asymmetry occur in patients who were asymmetrical to start with. I find it interesting that these patients often can be very demanding – they have high expectations of the procedure (see Markings).

Wound-healing Problems

See discussion on antibiotics and on gathering of the vertical incision under Operative Technique.

Loss of Sensation

When I switched away from the superior pedicle, I moved to a lateral pedicle because I thought that sensation would be better coming in from the lateral direction. But the shape was not as good because the base of the pedicle prevented adequate lateral resection. It was surprising to me that the sensation in the nipple was the same whether a superior, a lateral, or a medial pedicle was chosen. Eighty-five percent of patients maintained normal to near-normal sensation. I have not studied comparisons with the inferior pedicle, but my experience tells me that the sensation with all four pedicles is comparable – or nearly so.

Breastfeeding

I have had only 19 out of 1100 patients who subsequent to the surgery had a pregnancy. Thirteen were able to breastfeed and seven supplemented. Five patients were not able to breastfeed, and one did not try.

Dr. Norma Cruz-Korchin has studied breastfeeding in large-breasted women who came for a breast reduction consultation but who decided not to have surgery. She compared these patients with those who underwent a medial pedicle vertical breast reduction. Interestingly, she found that between 60 and 65 % of patients in both groups were able to breastfeed, and one quarter of these patients supplemented. Maternity nurses have often commented that it is the large-breasted women who seem to have trouble breastfeeding. Does the size of the breast contribute as much to the problem as the surgery itself?

Vertical Scar Mammaplasty with the Inferocentral Pedicle

Elisabeth Würinger

> **B**ehold, you are beautiful, my love,
>
> behold, you are beautiful!
>
> Your two breasts are like two fawns,
>
> twins of a gazelle,
>
> that feed among the lilies.
>
> *Song of Solomon 4.1, 4.5*

Introduction

Understanding the neurovascular supply along the ligamentous suspension has allowed the neurovascular supply in breast reduction procedures to be maintained more precisely. Only parts of this rich neurovascular supply are sufficient to nourish the nipple-carrying pedicle, thereby using one of the two main neurovascular sources, namely, a superficial dermal or a central, parenchymal path [4–7]. It is possible to combine those two main sources.

My technique derives its neurovascular supply by the horizontal septum within a central pedicle, which allows me to abandon all dermal connections. Taking advantage of the preexisting bipartition of the breast allows a blood-saving procedure and probably allows minimal risk of injury to the vessels, nerves, and lactiferous ducts. This approach to blunt resection can also be integrated into different reduction techniques like the inferior pedicle [1], in the course of which I found the horizontal septum. Even the principle of Hall-Findlay's technique [2], namely, rotating a medial pedicle upward, can be combined with the preservation of the horizontal septum.

Operative Technique

Markings

I usually mark the patient after sterile draping in a semiupright position (Fig. 8.1). The midsternal line and the inframammary fold are outlined, and the sternal notches at the jugulum and at the processus xiphoideus are marked as fix points. With the help of a mammary circle, all drawings are transferred symmetrically from one breast side to the other. The most important reference point is the marking of the new nipple site. I leave this point rather lower than the inframammary fold, especially in heavy, ptotic breasts. This point will be raised spontaneously when the distended skin shrinks, as soon as the heavy weight of the hypertrophic gland no longer pulls it down. More skin in the cranial part is necessary to cover a well-shaped breast after raising and shaping the gland than in a flat, ptotic breast. If the skin envelope in the upper parts of the breast gets too tight, the breast loses projection and the nipple may get too high. As in facial rejuvenation, ultimately the skin should cover rearranged structures without tension.

After determination of the new nipple site, the skin excess is determined by gently pulling the breast medially and laterally upward, where it crosses the vertical axis of the breast, similar to the technique of Lejour [3]. These vertical lines are joined cranially just below the marking of the new nipple position, caudally about 4–5 cm, in bigger breasts 6–8 cm above the submammary fold, as the submammary fold will be elevated. The lines finally build a periareolar circle or oval shape (Figs. 8.1, 8.2). Above this circle a very flat hemicircular line, just including the new nipple position, is drawn symmetrically on both the right and left breast. This line determines the presumptive new periareolar closure line, and its extent is planned in such a way that the skin excess is distributed roughly equally between the future periareolar and vertical scar. For more than 2 years I have been keeping a medial narrow dermal bridge of about 2–3 cm between the periareolar circle and the skin envelope, which is outlined symmetrically. The size of the areola is determined with an areola marker, and the areola is incised intracutaneously. In most cases my preferred size is 42 mm.

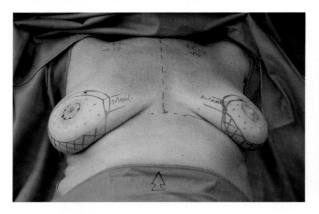

Fig. 8.1. Preoperative marking of the circular periareolar skin excess using a semiupright position. Deepithelialization is performed in the stippled area, and the skin in the stripped area is removed full thickness. The medial dermal bridge is marked *MED*. The *flat hemicircular line* includes the new nipple position

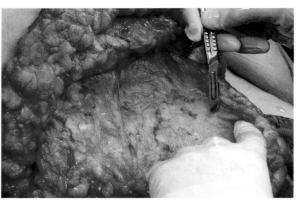

Fig. 8.3. After horizontal incision of the gland, which leaves the cranial part intact, the retromammary space is reached

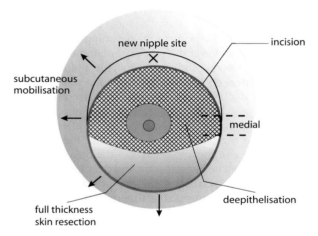

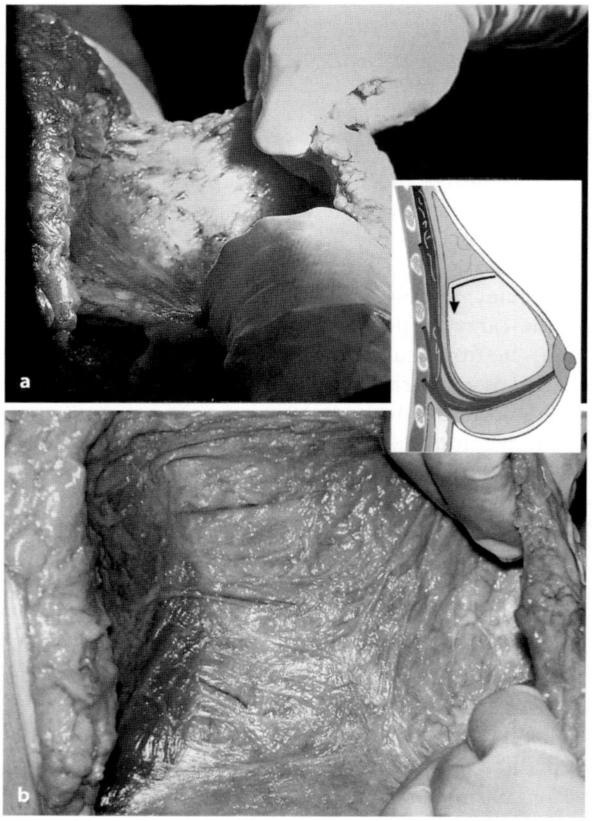

Fig. 8.2. Schematic diagram showing circular incision along the periareolar dermal ring (*red*) by maintaining a narrow medial dermal bridge (*blue*). Subcutaneous mobilization is limited to the lateral and caudal parts of the breast

Preparation

In the lateral and caudal region the skin envelope outside the periareolar circle is infiltrated with 0.5% xylocaine with epinephrine within the subcutaneous layer only. The cranial part and the future medial dermal bridge are not infiltrated. In small breasts all the periareolar excess skin circle is deepithelialized, which can be used to support the shape of the gland. In larger breasts only part of the periareolar dermal circle is deepithelialized, and the caudal part of the skin excess can be excised in full thickness (Figs. 8.1, 8.2). Then the remaining skin envelope is incised circularly on the peripheral side of the periareolar skin excess.

Fig. 8.4 a,b. *Insert:* The retromammary space is followed bluntly to the fourth intercostal space. Blunt resection opens up the areolar tissue in an anterior direction to the nipple. From [4], with permission of *Plastic Reconstructive Surgery*. **a** Blunt resection in a clinical breast reduction. **b** The same dissection in anatomical preparation showing the cranial vascular layer of the horizontal septum after intra-arterial injection of colored latex into the thoracoacromial artery. From [6], with permission of *European Journal of Morphology*

In the lateral and caudal region the skin envelope is separated from the gland in a thin subcutaneous plane to the thoracic wall. This subcutaneous plane in most cases can be found easily by gently pushing the open scissors forward parallel and about 2 cm below the skin. In the region of the submammary fold, I cautiously guide the dissection away from the pedicle. Recently, I used to keep the above-mentioned narrow dermal bridge between the deepithelialized circle and the skin envelope. This dermal bridge prevents the glandular pedicle from sinking too low, which happens after total isolation, and thereby fixation sutures can be economized. Cranially, the uppermost parts of the breast are left intact, thereby maintaining cranial fullness (Figs. 8.3, 8.4), and a horizontal incision goes through the gland to reach the retromammary space approximately at the level of the third rib, where a vascular layer gets faintly through.

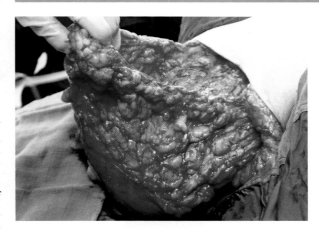

Fig. 8.5. Left breast lateral view: after blunt separation of the cranial glandular layer to the nipple, sharp resection of the vertical ligaments and along the cranial dermal ring follows

Resection

The resection of the residual cranial glandular layer is then performed. In this technique, advantage is taken of the preexisting bipartition of the breast. As soon as the retromammary space is reached, gentle, blunt finger dissection is used to follow the plane of areolar connective tissue down to the level of the fourth intercostal space. Here the retromammary space ends and merges into areolar tissue, which can be progressively opened up with the fingers in an anterior direction to the nipple, always staying above the horizontal septum (Fig. 8.4). Thus resection can largely be done by blunt dissection, following the gliding layer along the retromammary space, which continues on its course to the nipple.

As it approaches the nipple the areolar layer may get less distinct, and a little more forceful blunt finger dissection may be necessary to reach the horizontal plane behind the nipple. Also, the cranial and caudal layers of lactiferous ducts and sinuses are separated bluntly along the horizontal septum as far as the nipple. In this way the caudal layer of duct openings into the nipple can be maintained intact, which very probably preserves the possibility of breastfeeding postoperatively.

By blunt preparation to the medial and lateral sides, the vertical ligaments are encountered (Fig. 8.5). The vertical ligaments can be maintained or dissected sharply according to the desired breast size. If the medial dermal bridge is maintained, part of the medial ligament is also maintained. The lateral ligament and even the lateral third of the horizontal septum will usually be dissected. This dissection should leave some tissue at the origin of the horizontal septum to preserve the deep branch of the lateral cutaneous branch of the fourth intercostal nerve, which runs within the retromammary space from lateral to medial and changes direction after 3 to 5 cm to rise toward the nipple along the level of the fibrous septum [7]. In any case, all the cranial glandular layers above the horizontal septum, including the Tail of Spence, can be removed bluntly without any danger to this nerve branch. This allows for the resection of the lateral fullness, which often causes a broad-based and square-shaped breast.

After peeling off the cranial glandular layer, the pedicle consists finally of the horizontal fibrous septum and its attached neurovascular layers, as well as the caudal glandular layer (Fig. 8.6 a). If the medial dermal bridge is maintained, a second source of neurovascular supply is provided along the medial ligament including the vigorous perforating branches from anastomoses of the internal thoracic artery arising in the second and third intercostal spaces and the accompanying nerves (Fig. 8.6 b). Resection of the thin caudal glandular layer will rarely be necessary and should be performed carefully so as not to hurt the main nerve and the caudal vascular layer, which is not delineated as clearly toward the gland as it is on the cranial vascular layer [4,7].

At this stage of the procedure it is helpful to operate on the contralateral side up to the same step to achieve symmetry. The difference in volume in different sized breasts is caused mainly by the cranial glandular layer, which is largely removed in this technique. This allows for the removal of the very region where the actual hypertrophy and accumulation of fat seem to take place. The thickness of the pedicle, including the caudal glandular layer, will be equal on both sides [4]. Therefore, the horizontal septum can be used as a guide to achieve symmetry also in preoperatively asymmetric breasts. To obtain equal sizes, not only the pedicle but also the thickness of the skin envelope must be checked for symmetry.

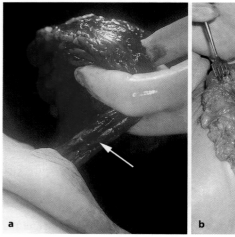

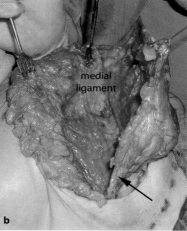

Fig. 8.6 a,b. After resection, the nipple-bearing central pedicle comprises the horizontal septum and the caudal glandular layer. **a** The pedicle (*arrow*) after complete isolation. After [4], with permission of *Plastic Reconstructive Surgery*. **b** If a medial dermal bridge is retained, part of the medial ligament is also maintained. The horizontal septum is seen from the lateral view (*arrow*)

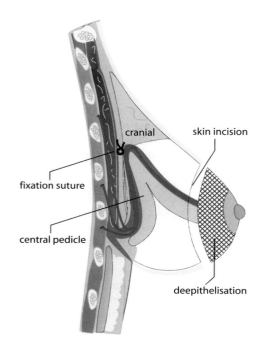

Fig. 8.7. Lateral view: after total isolation of the pedicle, the pedicle is translocated upward by fixation sutures. After [4], with permission of *Plastic Reconstructive Surgery*

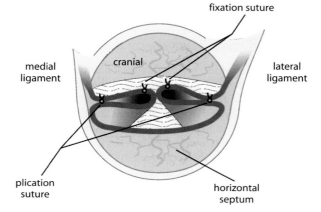

Fig. 8.8. Anterior view: the lateral ligaments can be shortened by plication and fixed to the thoracic wall. After [4], with permission of *Plastic Reconstructive Surgery*

Modeling

After resection, shaping of the breast cone follows. When the pedicle is totally isolated, fixation to the thoracic wall is necessary to raise the pedicle (Figs. 8.7, 8.8). Its fibrous elements provide sturdy structures for fixation, unlike the residual breast parenchyme, where sutures cut through easily. The rims of the horizontal septum or the vertical ligaments can be shortened by plication sutures, and the plicated part can be sus-

pended at the pectoralis fascia. This allows excellent modeling of the breast, which can be further supported by a dermal brassiere built by the periareolar skin excess, which in turn can be fixed to the thoracic wall. But all those sutures may irritate the neurovascular supply running along the ligamentous suspension and thus should be placed cautiously so as not to cause congestion.

This made me keep intact a medial dermal bridge of about 2 to 3 cm that holds the pedicle in a higher position. The medial dermal connection between the pedicle and the skin envelope, as well as the medial part of the horizontal septum, acts as a pivot point that allows the lateral edge of the pedicle comprising the horizontal septum to rotate upward, according to the principle of the Hall-Findlay technique [2]. Thus, far fewer or even no fixation sutures are necessary. In this way the advantage of a technique keeping the upper parts of the breast intact, which acts against the force of gravity, can be combined with the advantage of having an intact horizontal septum, which implicates an optimized neurovascular supply. In this way also a double source of neurovascular supply is provided both by the horizontal septum and the medial ligament.

Final Adjustment

After modeling the breast cone, the skin envelope is rearranged. The flat hemicircular line, which includes the new nipple position, is arranged around the nipple, and the two end points of this line are joined with a suture. In this way the skin excess is distributed more or less equally, half around the nipple, half caudal of the nipple into the vertical scar. At this stage the final skin resection is brought up to the final shape and size of the breast cone. Usually, skin is resected following the hemicircular line above the suture; sometimes all skin around the nipple will be maintained to provide sufficient projection. Contrary to the cranial part of the breast, where I leave generous amounts of skin, I remove any residual skin excess caudal of the nipple. Again, extensive tension must be avoided. The skin excess caudal of the suture can be estimated in a freehand style or by inverting it and stapling the plicated skin excess temporarily together. The redundant skin is resected and gathered in a two-layer closure, thereby reducing its length. As soon as the medial and lateral pillars are joined, improvement of projection and shape can be observed.

By no means should the vertical resection reach the inframammary fold. In case of more marked skin excess, the caudal end of the resection line is directed in a curve laterally, always staying 2 to 3 cm above the inframammary fold. In this case the mediocaudal skin edge is larger than the craniolateral edge and must be gathered equally to the shorter side. Where the skin resection interferes with the medial dermal bridge, deepithelialization is performed. Part of the skin excess is gathered around the nipple in a two-layer closure, with some Vicryl stitches distributing the skin equally. Skin closure is performed with partially intracutaneous nonresorbably single-knot

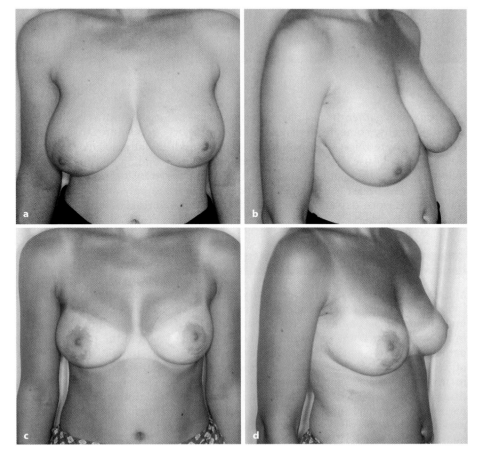

Fig. 8.9 a–d. Young patient with moderate hypertrophy and asymmetry before and 1 year after resection of 300 g on both right and left side (medial dermal bridge)

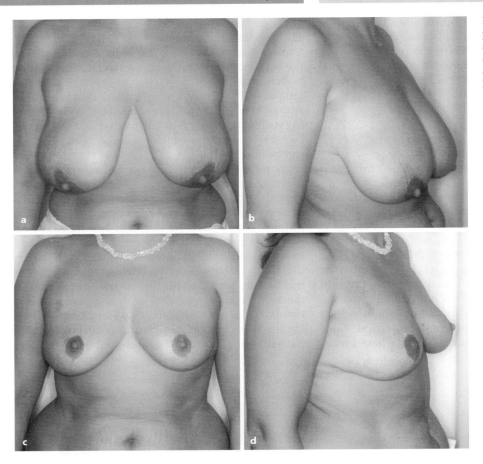

Fig. 8.10 a–d. Middle-aged patient with marked ptosis and hypertrophy before and 3 years after resection of 500 g on both right and left breast

stitches, which gather the peripheral periareolar skin excess. Initially, some fine wrinkles may be seen along the suture lines; these will settle after several weeks. I usually use drains, which are removed the following day; the patient stays at the hospital overnight. The breast is bandaged for 2 days. Then a sports bra is worn day and night, after 2 weeks only during the day.

Results

Maintaining sensibility, sexual sensitivity, and erectility of the nipple is a major concern of many women undergoing breast reduction. This could be secured in all cases after blunt resection. In more than 100 patients up to 2100 g per breast with an average weight of 720 g per side was resected. Neurovascular supply to the nipple-areola complex was optimized in all cases, as it was provided by the horizontal septum and parts of the vertical ligaments following blunt preparation. These fibrous structures, which guide the neurovascular supply, provide a high shaping poten-

tial but must be handled carefully when placing fixation sutures to avoid congestion. When the pedicle is totally isolated, a couple of fixation sutures and some folding of the pedicle are necessary for superior translocation of the pedicle. This did not irritate the supply of the nipple, but it did congest parts of the breast tissue in some patients. A certain vascular compromise indeed resulted in oil cysts in a few cases, which required punctation or even operative resection of fat necrosis. Since I first started applying Hall-Findlay's principle of rotating the pedicle upward, the need for fixation sutures has been drastically reduced and since that time no more congestion of breast tissue has occurred.

Maintaining the continuity of the lactiferous ducts within the intact caudal glandular layer likely favors postoperative lactation. In all cases of pregnancy (five patients), uncomplicated breastfeeding was possible. The breasts showed stable, conical shape (Figs. 8.9–8.12), and no significant settling was necessary to find the final breast shape. There is no marked difference between early and late appearance. The technique allows one to adjust the final breast size to the individ-

Fig. 8.11 a–d. Elderly, adipose patient before and 4 years after resection of 1360 g right breast and 1200 g left breast

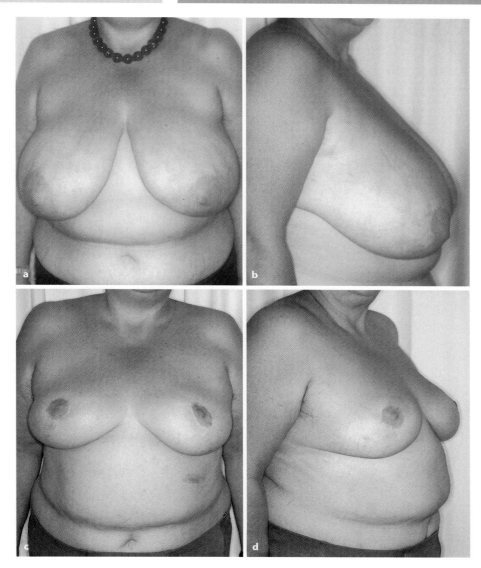

ual wishes of the patient, whether that means keeping the size rather large or small.

Significant superior translocation of the nipple is not limited by a dermal pedicle, nor is keeping the medial dermal bridge a limiting factor. The inframammary fold can be lifted, and there is no migration of the vertical scar below the inframammary fold. Underresection of skin can lead to a dog ear above the inframammary fold, which happened in two cases.

Even though no liposuction is performed, a higher percentage of neurovascular and fibrous tissue is present after resection of the hypertrophied and fatty cranial glandular layer. Future loss and gain of body weight after reduction will lead to less shape change because of less fat in the postoperative breast (Fig. 8.11). The vertical scar seems to be less a "punc-

tum minoris resistenciae" compared to the inverted T scar and tends to bottom out less.

Subcutaneous undermining of the skin is limited to the lateral and caudal region of the breast. Resection of the lateral part of the cranial glandular layer far up into the axilla results in a relatively long lateral skin flap, which carries a risk of necrosis at the junction with the perimamillar scar. This occurred in two patients. Apart from maintaining the tender neurovascular network within the immediate periareolar dermis, deepithelialization is not important for the supply of the nipple and can be limited to a minimum. Nevertheless, I prefer to keep a certain amount of dermis, which allows some modeling of the breast shape.

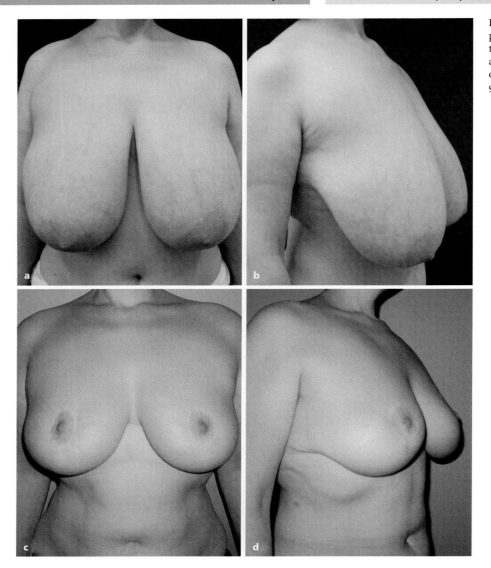

Fig. 8.12 a–d. Middle-aged patient with marked hypertrophy and ptosis before and 3 years after resection of 870 g on right breast and 940 g on left breast

As a result of gathering the skin excess, both the periareolar scar and the vertical scar reduce skin wrinkling, the wrinkling is distributed equally along the whole extent of the scar line, and thereby represents a combination of both the purse-string and vertical techniques. Additionally, the safety and familiarity of the inferior pedicle, from which my technique developed, can be combined with the static advantage of an upward rotation of the pedicle.

References

1. Georgiade NG, Serafin D, Riefkohl R, Georgiade GS (1979) Is there a reduction mammaplasty for "all seasons?" Plast Reconstr Surg 63:165

2. Hall-Findlay EJ (1999) A simplified vertical reduction mammaplasty: shortening the learning curve. Plast Reconstr Surg 104:748

3. Lejour M (1994) Vertical mammaplasty and liposuction of the breast. Plast Reconstr Surg 94:100

4. Würinger E (1999) Refinement of the central pedicle breast reduction by application of the ligamentous suspension. Plast Reconstr Surg 103:1400

5. Würinger E (2002) Secondary reduction mammaplasty. Plast Reconstr Surg 109:812

6. Würinger E, Tschabitscher M (2003) New aspects of the topography of the mammary gland regarding its neurovascular supply along a regular ligamentous suspension. Eur J Morphol 40(3):181

7. Würinger E, Mader N, Posch E, Holle J (1998) Nerve and vessel supplying ligamentous suspension of the mammary gland. Plast Reconstr Surg 101:1486

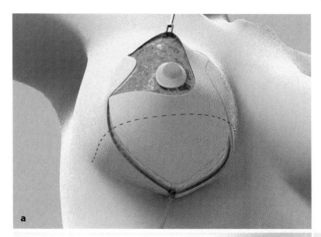

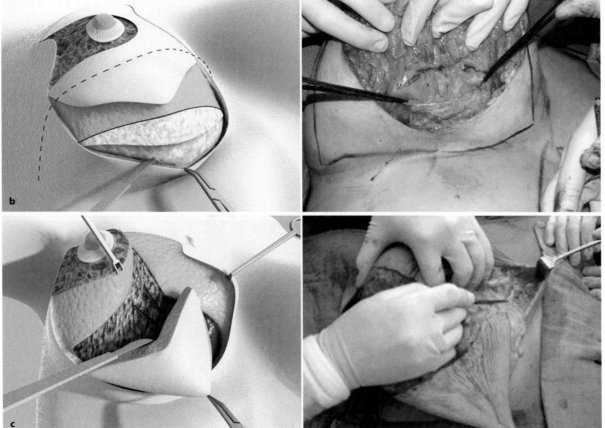

Fig. 9.3. **a** Deepithelialized pedicle and undermining of the skin over the lower pole of breast. **b** Dissection of superficial fascia 1–2 cm above IMF. **c** Resection of inferior pole

Surgical Procedure

The surgery is performed under general anesthesia with a local infiltration of the surgical lines and of the base of the breast with 40 cc 1% xylocaine with 1:80,000 adrenaline diluted with 40 cc saline. The pedicle itself is not infiltrated. The nipple-areola complex (NAC) is marked with a 4-cm-diameter areola marker without tension. The pedicle is deepithelialized, leaving 1.5 cm of dermis around the NAC.

The inferior pole of the breast skin is undermined, starting at 6 cm of each vertical line until 1 to 2 cm above the IMF (Fig. 9.3a). The thickness of the skin flap is similar to that of a postmastectomy skin. The superficial fascia is incised and dissected over the gland 2 cm above the IMF (Fig. 9.3b). This fascia is kept attached to the IMF and will be used to suspend

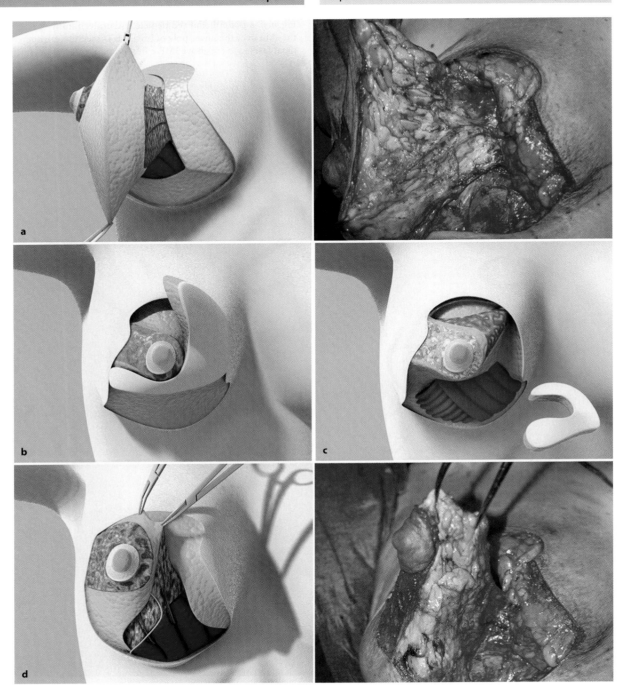

Fig. 9.4 a–d. The surgical technique in septum-based lateral mammaplasty. **a** The breast incised medially and cranially according to drawing lines. **b** C-shape resection of gland around pedicle. **c** Lateral pedicle still attached to thoracic wall by sep-tum. **d** The pedicle, which contains the intercostal perforators and nerves in addition to the deep branch of the fourth intercostal nerve, is rotated medially and cranially

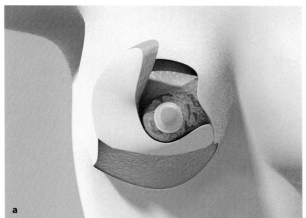

Fig. 9.5 a–c. The surgical technique in septum-based medial mammaplasty. **a** Breast is incised from cranial to lateral direction. **b** C-gland rescection around the pedicle. **c** V resection through septum; the medial pedicle is still attached to the thoracic wall by the septum, which contains some perforators and the deep branch of the fourth intercostal nerve

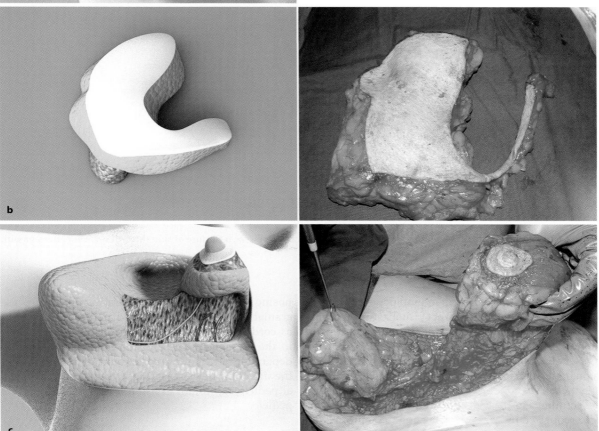

the IMF in a higher position at the end of the procedure. Then the resection of the inferior pole of the breast is continued through an almost nonvascular plane with the surgical knife. The incision begins at 6 cm from the base of the mosque-shaped design. The gland will peel off easily from the horizontal septum (Fig. 9.3c). Perforators and nerves can be seen and palpated as small cords incorporated within the septum.

Septum-based Lateral Pedicle (SLM)

The gland is first incised at the medial side to the pectoralis major (PM) fascia and then extended cranially until the base of the pedicle. With this incision the septum is cut at the medial side, and the vessels within are easily seen (Fig. 9.4a). Consequently, the pedicle is separated from the rest of the breast except for the lateral and central attachments. The resection is per-

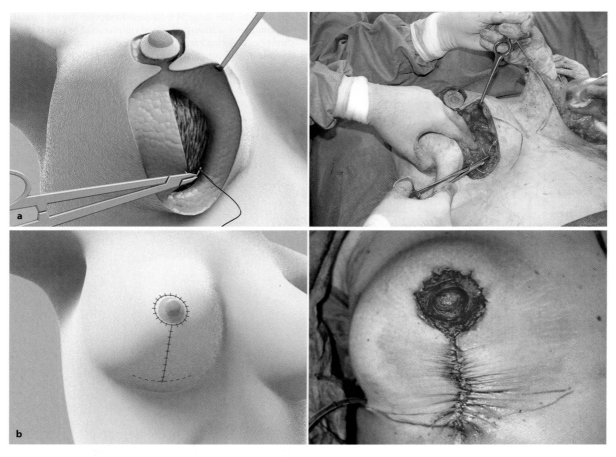

Fig. 9.6 a,b. Closure of breast. **a** Fixation of lateral pillar onto pectoralis fascia. **b** Closure of skin through vertical pattern or with short inverted T scar (optional)

formed around the pedicle in monobloc, and the pedicle can be sculpted under direct visualization and palpation of the horizontal septum. The main resection is done in the medial, superior, and central parts with preservation of the septum but with very limited excision in the inferior part of the pedicle to avoid damaging the nerves and the vessels included in the horizontal septum (Fig. 9.4 b). The resection is tailored to the size requested by the patient, leaving the septum connected to the thoracic wall (Fig. 9.4 c). The dermis of the pedicle is carefully incised at the base to allow better upward rotation (Fig. 9.4 d).

Septum-based Medial Pedicle (SMM)

In this case, the gland is incised first around the pedicle cranially to laterally, and then a V resection through the septum is performed under direct vision (Fig. 9.5 a). The vessels accompanied by the nerves can be identified through the septum by ex-

posing the septum to the operative light from the cranial side so the vessels and nerves can be seen as cords that run toward the pedicle like the vessels in the mesentery. The excision is extended laterally depending on the desired amount of resection and the size of the new breast (Fig. 9.5 b, c). As for the lateral pedicle, minimum excision is done distally to the pedicle.

Closure of the Breast. Meticulous hemostasis is performed. A 3–0 absorbable suture is used to close the top of the vertical pillars. The IMF is suspended and fixed onto the pectoralis fascia with heavy stitches using the superficial fascia, which was dissected at the beginning of the procedure. The lateral pillar is rotated medially and cranially and then strongly fixed to the pectoralis fascia by a few absorbable heavy polydixonan 1–0 stitches (Fig. 9.6 a). This leads to positioning of the pedicle centrally at its new location without tension. The pedicle is not fixed to the superior breast pole. Four cardinal 3–0 suture points are

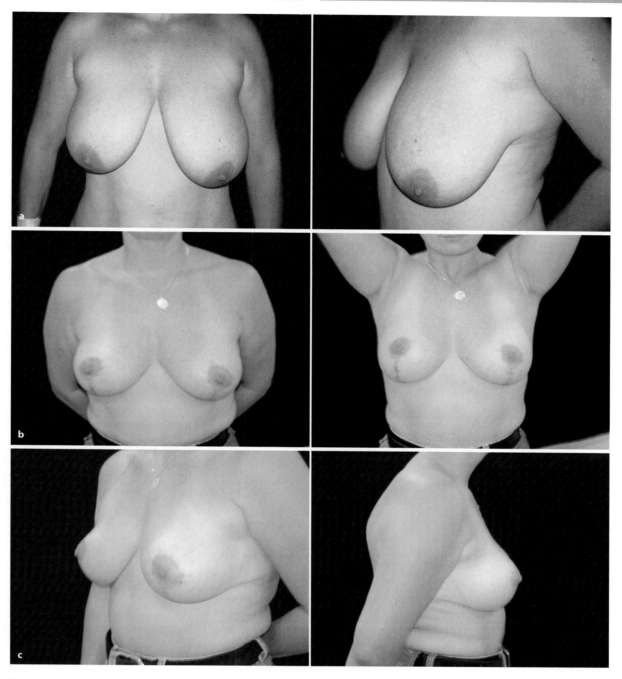

Fig. 9.7 a–c. A 30-year-old patient who had 380 g and 420 g of gland resection from the right and left breast, respectively. The nipple was 35 cm preoperatively and elevated to 22 cm from the sternal notch. **a** Preoperative views. **b, c** Postoperative views

placed on the deep dermis of the areola and extended to the dermis of the surrounding skin. A few polydiaxonan 1–0 stitches are used to bring the lateral and medial pillars together.

Depending on many factors such as skin quality, age of patient, smoking history, or patient wishes, the decision is made to close the breast with a vertical scar only or short L or inverted T pattern. If the vertical scar is opted for, the skin will be undermined to a limited extension so as to permit closure with small wrinkles (Fig. 9.6 b). Skin closure is done in two layers using interrupted 3–0 polydiaxonan on the deep dermis and running subcuticular 4–0 Monocryl on the skin.

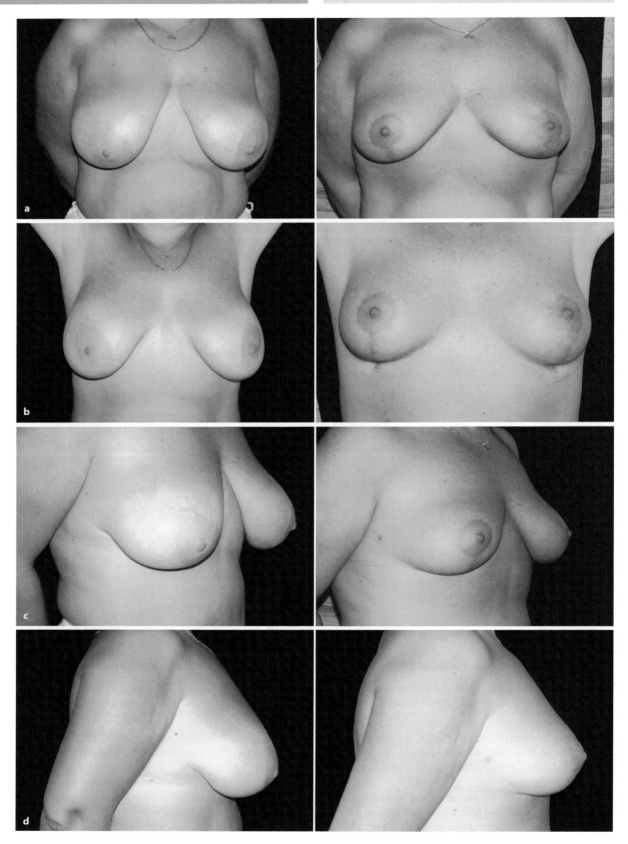

Fig. 9.8 a–d.

Fig. 9.8 a–d. Preoperative and postoperative views of a mildly overweight 35-year-old patient who had 376 g and 406 g removed from the right and left breast, respectively, to obtain the requested results, which fits her body

Postoperative Care

One suction drain is left in place in each breast. Attention must be paid to placing the drain behind the areola to avoid a retroareolar hematoma. A gauze dressing is used to cover the incisions, and a surgical brassiere is put on. The drains are removed after 1–2 days, and patients are discharged from the hospital. They are instructed to wear a sports bra night and day for 1 month.

Results

Since January 2000, 80 patients have undergone breast reduction using a septum-based mammaplasty. The pedicle for the nipple-areola complex is based on a horizontal septum and is designed to incorporate the lateral branch of the fourth intercostal vessels and of the nerve. Breasts with a 45-cm nipple-to-sternum notch were operated successfully using the septum-based pedicle technique. Mean gland resection was 580 g (40 to 1980 g) per breast. Septum-based lateral mammaplasty was the most used (80%). I currently use the septum-based medial mammaplasty with increasing frequency. Clinical cases are shown in Figs. 9.7–9.9. Choice between the two pedicles is discussed in Chap. 10.

Complications

The complication rate is obviously related to the learning curve. Most of the complications occurred in the first 15 patients, in particular wound dehiscence in case of significant breast hypertrophy. However, the areola was congested in one of my last patients, so leeches were applied on the areola. An extensive infection unexpectedly developed after a few days, probably due to the leeches, and led to a major necrosis of the central part of the breast with the NAC. The patient had a high risk factor – she was diabetic and a smoker with a ptosis of 38 cm – but I believe this kind of complication can occur in almost any patient, and no technique is spared such an extremely annoying problem. A retroareolar hematoma occurred at the beginning of our experience and resulted in a partial areola necrosis in one breast. Careful hemostasis and drain placement behind the NAC will prevent this complication.

Discussion

It is very difficult to invent a new technique in plastic surgery nowadays. "Something new is something old that has been forgotten," so we still adopt old ideas in order to improve them to incorporate them into our contemporary techniques. Skoog was the first to describe the lateral dermoglandular pedicle [12]. The concept of pedicle rotation medially [4, 13–14] or laterally in breast reduction has been reported by many authors [12,15,16]. However, these authors have not relied on determined anatomical structures for their techniques. The septum-based mammaplasty is an evolution of the lateral and medial pedicle techniques to improve sensitivity of NAC after reduction mammaplasty and to enhance blood supply to the pedicle by preserving the intercostal perforators in the septum. Many authors recommend minimal skin undermining [4, 6, 17]. Therefore, I have adopted a technique that maintains the attachment of the gland onto the overlying skin through the superficial fascial system [8] without separating the skin from the gland. This technique provides the required cone shape without the aspect of the high overprojected breast in the early postoperative period as occurred after Lassus's or Lejour's vertical mammaplasty due to the folded superior pedicle. One of the advantages of this technique is that the septum-based pedicle still allows a central gland resection while allowing the pedicle to remain attached to the thorax with the septum, which contains perforator vessels and nerves. Avoiding an inferior pedicle may avoid sagging and insure good breast projection.

In addition, the major advantage of the septum-based pedicle technique is that the integrity of the gland under the NAC is preserved. Therefore, this technique provides better NAC sensitivity by including the deep branch of the fourth intercostal nerve within the pedicle. We showed, by a prospective thorough evaluation [19], that the sensitivity of the NAC was preserved in the immediate postoperative period after a reduction mammaplasty based on the horizontal septum.

Based on a well-vascularized and constant anatomical structure such as the horizontal septum, the pedicle is safer, especially in the case of significant breast hypertrophy. The septum-based mammaplasty technique shows clear advantages over the conventional techniques of breast reduction in terms of ease of pedicle shaping and modeling in addition to NAC sensation and breastfeeding.

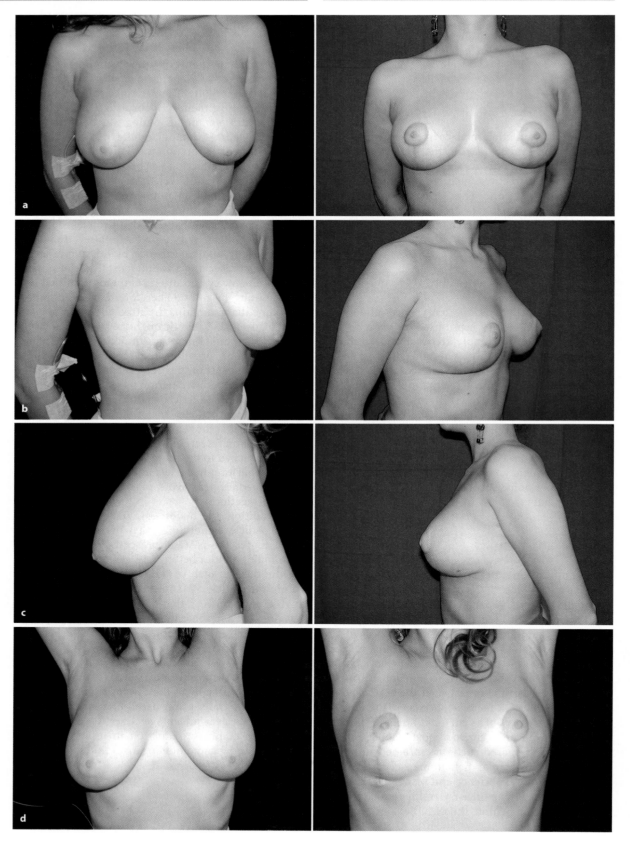

Fig. 9.9 a–d.

Fig. 9.9 a–d. Preoperative and postoperative views of an 18-year-old patient who had a gland resection of 360 and 350 g from right and left breast, respectively. She asked for mild reduction in order to give her the ability to breastfeed in the future

References

1. Arie G (1957) Una nueva tecnica de mastoplastia. Rev Iber Latino Am Cir Plast 3:28
2. Lassus C (1972) A new technique for breast reduction. Int Surg 53:69
3. Lejour M (1994) Vertical mammaplasty and liposuction of the breast. Plast Reconstr Surg 94:100
4. Hall-Findlay EJ (1999) A simplified vertical reduction mammaplasty: shortening the learning curve. Plast Reconstr Surg 104:748
5. Hammond DC (1999) Short scar periareolar inferior pedicle reduction (SPAIR) mammaplasty. Plast Reconstr Surg 103:890
6. Lassus C (1996) A 30-year experience with vertical mammaplasty. Plast Reconstr Surg 97:373
7. Lejour M (1999) Vertical mammaplasty: update and appraisal of late results. Plast Reconstr Surg 104:771
8. Hamdi M, Greuse M, DeMey A, Webster MHC (1999) Breast sensation after superior pedicle versus inferior pedicle mammaplasty: prospective clinical evaluation. Br J Plast Surg 54:39
9. Greuse M, Hamdi M, DeMey A (2001) Breast sensitivity after vertical mammaplasty. Plast Reconstr Surg 107:970
10. Würinger E, Mader N, Posch E, Holle J (1998) Nerve and vessel supplying ligamentous suspension of the mammary gland. Plast Reconstr Surg 101:1486
11. Schlenz I, Kuzbari R, Gruber H, Holle J (2000) The sensitivity of the nipple-areola complex: an anatomic study. Plast Reconstr Surg 105:905
12. Skoog T (1974) Plastic Surgery: New Methods and Refinements. Almquist and Wiksell, Stockholm
13. Asplund OA, Davies DM (1996) Vertical scar breast reduction with medial flap or glandular transposition of the nipple-areola. Br J Plast Surg 49:507
14. Beer GM, Morgenthaler W, Spicher I, Meyer VE (2001) Modifications in vertical scar breast reduction. Br J Plast Surg 54:341
15. Cardenas-Camerena L, Vergara R (2001) Reduction mammaplasry with superolateral dermoglandular pedicle: another alternative. Plast Reconstr Surg 107:693
16. Blondeel PN, Hamdi M, Van de Sijpe KA, Van Landuyt KH, Thiessen FE, Monstrey SJ (2003) The latero-central glandular pedicle technique for breast reduction. Br J Plast Surg 56:348
17. Ramirez OM (2002) Reduction mammaplasty with the "owl" incision and no undermining. Plast Reconstr Surg 109:512
18. Lockwood T (1999) Reduction mammaplasty and mastopexy with superficial fascial system suspension. Plast Reconstr Surg 103:1411
19. Hamdi M, Van de Sijpe K, Van Landuyt K, Blondeel PN, Monstrey S (2003) Evaluation of nipple-areola complex sensitivity after the latero-central glandular pedicle technique in breast reduction. Br J Plast Surg 56:360

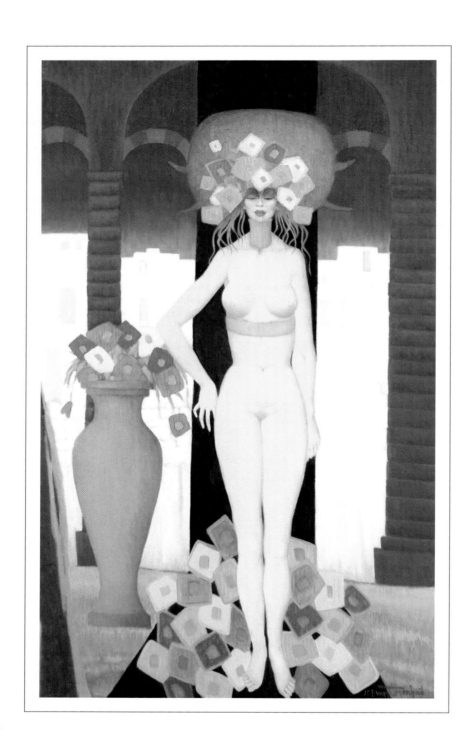

Different Approaches for Different Breasts

Claudio Cardoso de Castro, Sheyla Maria Carvalho Rodrigues

> **B**reasts are the symbol of a woman's femininity. The possibility of restoring a breast's form is a gift God gave to man.
>
> *Claudio Cardoso de Castro*

Techniques for breast reduction and mastopexy have evolved, as have philosophical concepts. The goal of a mastopexy or a reduction mammaplasty is to achieve breasts with pleasant appearance and firm, adequate size and form with minimal scarring and low rate of complications. Lactation and sexual functions must be preserved. If performed properly, the results are long lasting. The reason women demand aesthetic plastic surgery on their breasts is that they dislike aspects related to their appearance such as volume, shape, or consistency. Patients who undergo a reduction mammaplasty or mastopexy know beforehand that there will be a scar after the surgery. Every breast is different; therefore, every operation is different, and so the scars are different, in quality and appearance, regardless of length. It is the appearance of the scar that matters, not its length.

Planning the Mammaplasty

When breasts are assessed, it is noticed that there are some similarities between the two breasts, but no two breasts are identical. The volume and consistency of breast tissue, the grade of ptosis, the position of the nipple-areola complex in relation to the breast, and the distance of the nipples from the sternal notch vary so much that it is impossible to make an acceptable classification grouping every breast. Every technique for breast reduction or mastopexy requires skin resection and tissue removal. Due to the variations, one cannot apply the same type of skin resection or tissue removal to every patient.

When planning a mammaplasty, many factors must be taken into consideration: (a) breast size and consistency, (b) grade of ptosis, (c) distance between the suprasternal notch and nipples, (d) location of the nipple on the breast, (e) skin quality, and, most important, (f) the relationship between breast tissue and skin. Depending on these factors, it is our opinion that each breast deserves individualized skin markings [1] (not patterns) and individualized tissue resection. In sum, the greater the skin excess in relation to the breast tissue, the more skin will be removed. The amount of skin resected determines the length of the scar. When one tries to reduce the length of the scar by limiting skin removal, the form and appearance of the breasts are usually compromised. In this chapter, first skin markings are discussed, and then the different methods of tissue removal are described.

Skin Resection

First a line is drawn from the midclavicle to the submammary sulcus passing through the nipple. At the projection of this line, a point is marked on the submammary fold. This point, A, corresponds to the new position of the nipple-areola complex. It can be placed lower in some cases when the breast tissue is firm and the surgeon notices that lifting the nipples will be difficult. Sometimes it is easier to elevate the nipple and areola several centimeters and sometimes even 2 cm is very difficult (Figs. 10.1.1–10.1.2). After determining the position of point A, the most important maneuver is then performed. This is the positioning of points B and C (Figs. 10.1.3, 10.1.4). The definition of these points depends on the relationship between skin and breast tissue, as well as on the surgeon's skill, experience, and common sense. Points B and C define the new form and consistency of the "new breast." They should not be more than 7 cm from point A because if these lines are too long, the distance from the lower extremity of the areola to the submammary fold, which tends to elongate, will be too long and the appearance of the breasts will be not good in the long term. These lines can be more or less curved depending on the skin excess [2]. The greater the skin excess, the more curved the lines AB–AC should be. Points B and C are then linked to the lateral and medial extremities of the inframammary fold.

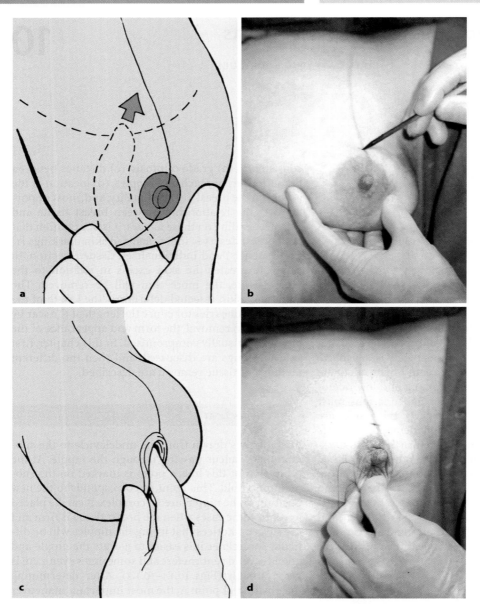

Fig. 10.1 a–d. Representation of the marking of points.
a Schematic representation of the marking of point A.
b Preoperative view.
c Evaluating the location of points B and C.
d Preoperative view

The extension of the inframammary incision depends on the size of the breast and chiefly on the relationship between skin and breast tissue. If there is skin excess, this excess must be eliminated. The final scar may be long, but if the skin excess is not treated in order to minimize the scar, the end result will certainly not be good. One must avoid joining the incision in the median line.

If the patient presents a mild hypertrophy and good skin quality, a vertical scar with or without a small compensation in the inframammary fold is recommended. These markings must be made in such a way that the final sutures are without tension of any

kind. The sutures without tension yield inconspicuous scars regardless of length.

With these principles (Pitanguy's [3–4] principles) in mind, basically we have three different types of skin markings as well as three different types of final scars (Figs. 10.2.1–10.2.4): (a) classic inverted T, (b) inverted T with a small horizontal scar at the inframammary fold, and (c) vertical scar. All these techniques leave a periareolar and a vertical scar. The appearance of these scars will vary according to each individual patient. I have used the periareolar approach [5] for selected cases (mild hypertrophy with good skin quality and with no ptosis). As the indications for the

Fig. 10.2 a–d. Types of skin markings. **a** Three different types of skin markings. **b** Classic inverted T. **c** Vertical scar. **d** Inverted T with small compensation of the inframammary fold

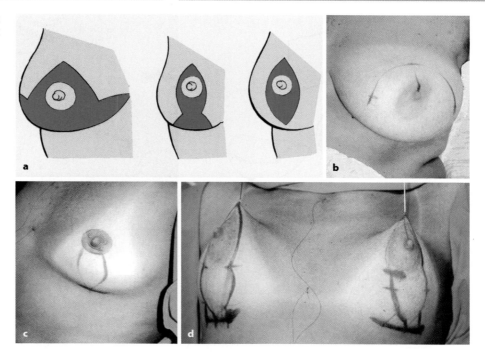

periareolar technique are uncommon, this procedure is not discussed in this chapter.

Tissue Resection

The type of tissue resection depends on the size, consistency, and form of the breast and mainly on the relationship between breast tissue and skin. I have been using three different types of breast tissue resection: (a) plane resection [6], (b) posterior resection [6], and (c) keel resection [3] (Figs. 10.3.1–10.3.6). I recommend the plane resection for hypertrophies where the superior pole is flat. The patient needs her breasts reduced but requires tissue in the upper pole (Figs. 10.3.1, 10.3.2). The posterior resection produces nice results in hypertrophy with excess tissue in the superior pole and in addition allows removal of a large amount of tissue (Figs. 10.3.3, 10.3.4). The keel resection, in my opinion, is the best option for an overall breast reduction (Figs. 10.3.5, 10.3.6).

Discussion

Currently there is a tendency among surgeons to reduce the final scar of a mammaplasty [7–11]. Plastic surgeons always avoid creating a long scar in any kind of operation. When a woman demands breast surgery, she desires to improve her appearance regardless of scars. I have had no complaints concerning

the extension of the scar but many concerning the quality and appearance of the scar. Sometimes patients complain about the size or form of their breasts. If it is necessary to increase the extension of the scar to improve the appearance of the breast, all patients agree with this course of action. Every breast has the scar it deserves.

In the service of plastic surgery of the Hospital of the University of the State of Rio de Janeiro, more than 4000 breast reductions and mastopexies were performed from 1974 to 2001. The level of satisfaction as well as complications has been low. I do believe that Pitanguy's [3–4] principles are the state of the art in mastopexy and reduction mammaplasty so far. These principles are simple, reliable, easy to learn, and applicable to every type of breast (Figs. 10.4–10.8).

Conclusion

Ongoing studies concerning level of satisfaction and complications, as well as evaluation of short-term and long-term results and patient opinion [12], allow me to assert that the final aspect of the breasts is the most important issue in breast reduction or mastopexy, regardless of the length of the scar (if the quality is good). Patients are concerned with scar quality, not with the extension of the scar. The patient must be totally pleased with the outcome of the surgery regardless of the technique used and the extension of the scar.

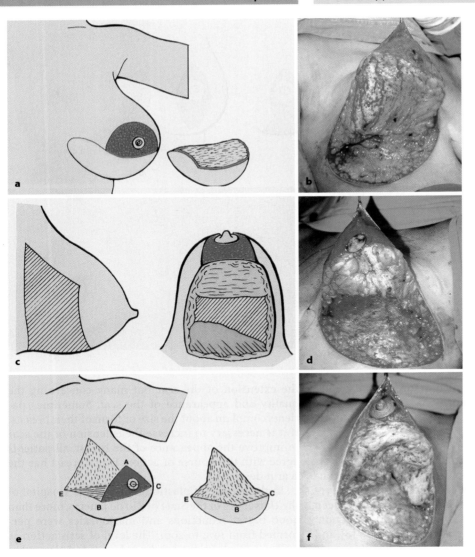

Fig. 10.3 a–f. Represen-
tation of the tissue
resection.
a Plane resection.
b Operative view.
c Posterior resection.
d Operative view.
e Keel resection.
f Operative view

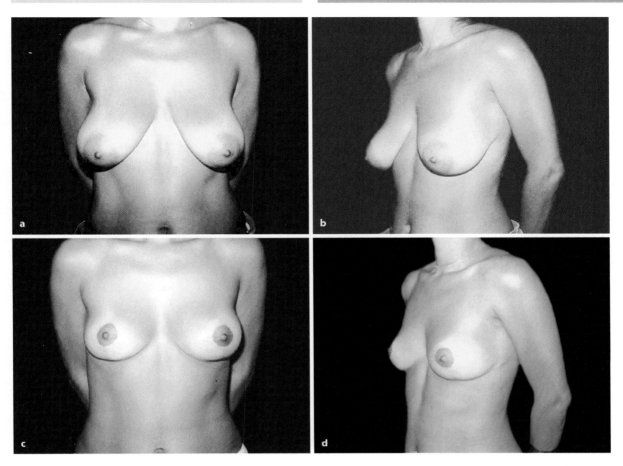

Fig. 10.4 a, b. Preoperative view of a patient with mammary ptosis. There is no tissue on the upper mammary pole. Voluminous skin excesses. **c, d** One year after mastopexy. Only skin was removed. No scars are visible

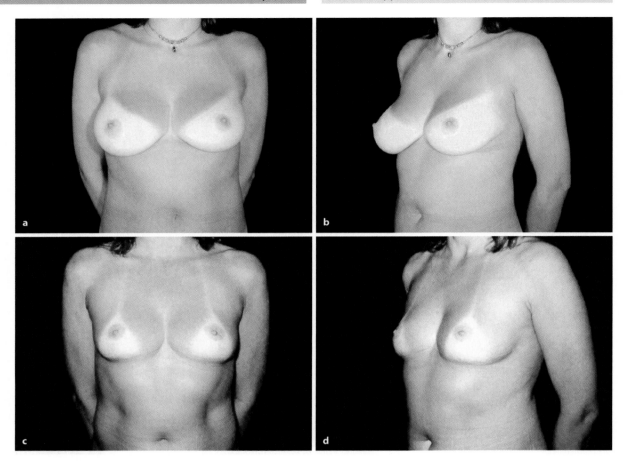

Fig. 10.5 a, b. Preoperative appearance of a patient demanding reduction mammaplasty complaining about discomfort due to the size of her breasts. **c, d** Appearance 8 years after reduction mammaplasty. During this period the patient had a baby. She breastfed normally. Form, size, and consistence were preserved

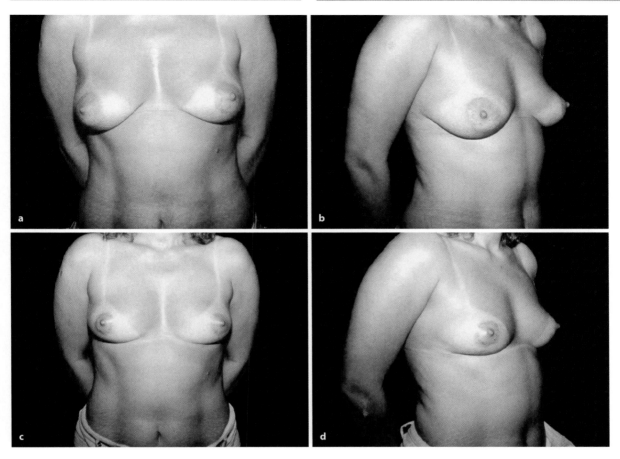

Fig. 10.6 a, b. Patient with mild hypertrophy, good skin quality. **c, d** Six months after mastopexy. Vertical scar and reduced scar in the submammary fold

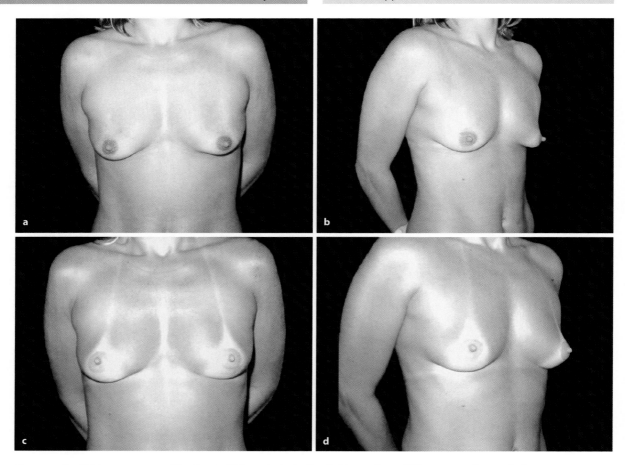

Fig. 10.7 a, b. Thirty-seven-year-old patient with breast ptosis. Good skin quality. **c, d** Three years after vertical mastopexy

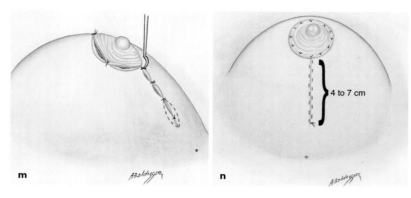

m   n

Fig. 11.1. a The new areola is outlined with a 3.5-cm diameter. **b** Points B and C are marked by pinching the skin at the level of the nipple and seeing the amount of resectable skin in the horizontal plane. The position of point A is confirmed by the projection of the upper pole over the submammary sulcus. **c** Point D is marked 3.0 cm above the submammary sulcus and 10.0 cm from the xiphoid appendix. Points A–D are joined in curved and straight ways, achieving a lozenge-shaped outline. **d** The inferior based pedicle is outlined. **e** Deepithelialization within the markings. **f** A horizontal incision is made below the areola and carried down to the pectoralis fascia. **g** After undermining of the inferior pole the inferior pedicle is created. **h** Resection of lateral and medial prolongations. **i** Following completion of inferior pedicle and resection of gland of upper pole of breast. **j** Fixation of pedicle on pectoralis fascia. **k** The closure of the breast is begun by closing the vertical incision until it is 4 to 7 cm from point D, depending on the size of the breast. **l** Checking for the presence of excess of skin. **m** The dog ear to be excised is marked. **n** Areola and vertical suturing is completed. Vertical scar does not extend beyond submammary fold

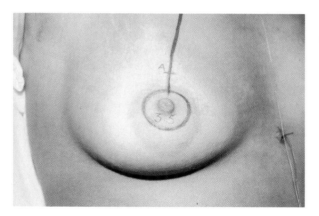

Fig. 11.2. The new areola is outlined with a 3.5-cm diameter

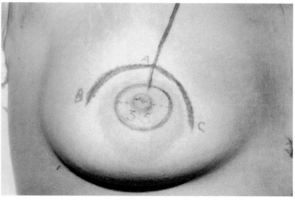

Fig. 11.3. Points A, B, and C are marked and joined with a curved line

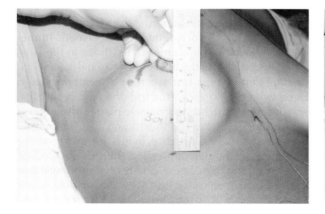

Fig. 11.4. Point D is marked 3.0 cm above the submammary fold on the meridian line of the breast

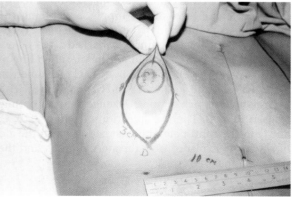

Fig. 11.5. Points B, D, and C are joined with straight lines, producing a lozenge-shaped outline, hence the designation "lozenge technique." Point D is located approximately 10.0 cm from the xiphoid appendix

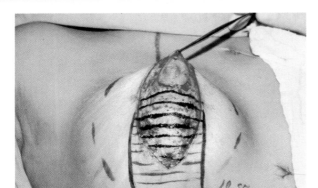

Fig. 11.6. Deepithelialization of the lozenge area and marking of the inferiorly based pedicle

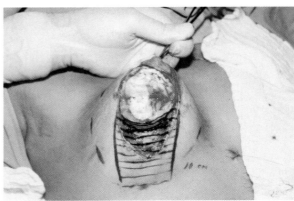

Fig. 11.7. Elaboration of the inferior pedicle begins with a horizontal incision made immediately below the areola

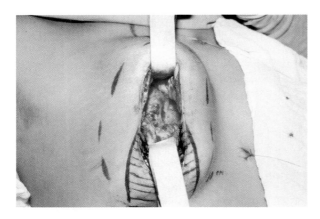

Fig. 11.8. The incision is carried down to the pectoralis fascia dividing the breast into two halves

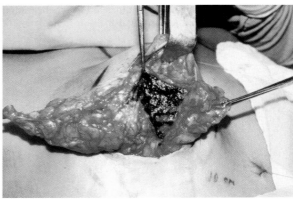

Fig. 11.9. The whole inferior pole of the breast is freed

ously drawn line. This becomes the future upper level of the areola. Points B and C are marked by pinching the skin, at the level of the nipple, and seeing the amount of excisable skin in the horizontal plane (Figs. 11.1b, 11.3). And, finally, point D is marked 2.5 to 3.0 cm above the submammary fold on the meridian line of the breast (Fig. 11.4). Points AB and AC are joined in a curved way, and points BD and CD are joined with a straight line, achieving a lozenge-shaped outline (Figs. 11.1c, 11.5). The transposition of points A, B, C, and D to the contralateral breast is done with the aid of suture lines placed over the sternal notch and the xiphoid appendix.

The Operation

The skin is deepithelialized within the markings (Figs. 11.1e, 11.6). A horizontal incision is made immediately below the areola and carried down to the muscular layer dividing the breast into two halves, superior and inferior (Figs. 11.1f, 11.7, 11.8). The inferior half is freed from the skin with the use of a pair of scissors, leaving it attached to the muscle plane, while one is careful not to injure the fourth and fifth intercostal perforating vessels, which provide the nutrition for this dermoglandular flap called the inferior pedicle (Figs. 11.1g, 11.9). The lateral and medial prolongations of the flap are resected (Fig. 11.1h). The pedicle is now complete and will be transposed to the upper pole and fixed to the pectoralis fascia, giving the breast a more conical shape and long-lasting result.

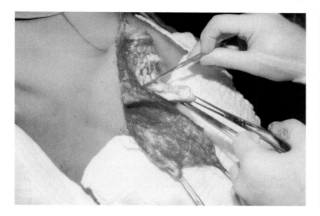

Fig. 11.10. The inferiorly based pedicle is formed after resection of the lateral and medial segments. Excess of mammary tissue is resected from the central area of the superior pole until it reaches the desired size

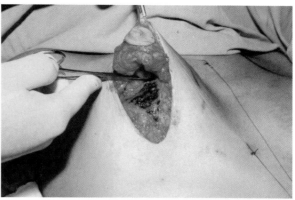

Fig. 11.11. The pedicle is left to drop naturally over the pectoralis fascia and fixed with nonabsorbable sutures

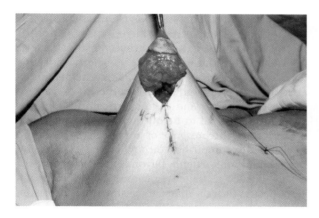

Fig. 11.12. With the entire upper pole pulled upwards, closing the breast starts by joining edge BD to CD with sutures from point D until it is 4 to 7 cm from it. The areola is sutured in such a way as to compensate for the excess skin

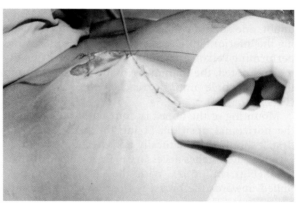

Fig. 11.13. It is important to check for the presence of skin excess in the inferior end of the incision

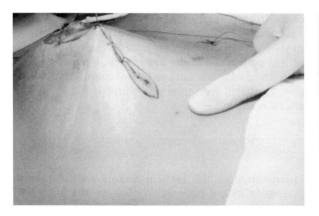

Fig. 11.14. The excess is marked, and care should be taken not to extend the line of resection beyond the submammary fold

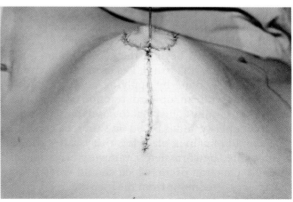

Fig. 11.15. End result. Areola and vertical suturing is completed. The vertical scar does not extend beyond the submammary fold

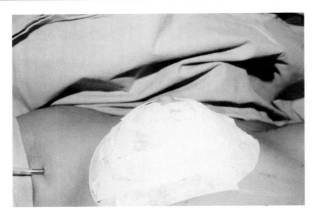

Fig. 11.16. Final immobilization with microporous adhesive tape, which should remain in place for 10 days

At this point it is important to check the vascularization of the flap that has been created. If there is any doubt, one should change the surgical plan, discarding the inferior flap, leaving the upper pole intact, and performing Peixoto's technique. If no vascular impairment is noted, the mammary tissue is resected from the upper pole until it reaches the desired size (Figs. 11.1i, 11.10).

Mounting of the breast is done with the patient in the horizontal position. Fixing the pedicle is done first. It should drop naturally, and the number and location of the stitches necessary to fix it will vary by patient (Figs. 11.1j, 11.11). With the entire upper pole pulled upwards the breast is closed, joining the skin edge BD to CD and making the vertical incision. The suture starts from point D and goes until it is 4 to 7 cm from it, depending on the size of the breast (Figs. 11.1k, 11.12). The nipple-areola complex is sutured in such a way as to compensate for the excess skin. No skin resection is required.

A hook should be placed at the junction of the vertical incision to the areola and pulled upwards. In most instances, a dog ear is present in the inferior part of the vertical incision and must be excised, taking care not to extend beyond the submammary sulcus (Figs. 11.1l, 11.1m, 11.13–11.15). The breast is then immobilized. This is done by applying adhesive microporous tape with an upward traction of the breast (Fig. 11.16). It is the equivalent to nasal immobilization after rhinoplasty and is based on skin retraction. The tape should remain in place for 10 days, after which it is substituted by a brassiere. Drainage is accomplished through a suction drain, which should emerge from the axillary area, never from the incision.

Complications

Necrosis

Since we started using this technique we have had no instances of total or partial necrosis of the nipple-areola complex, no skin or fat necrosis, and no atrophy of the pedicle.

Sensation

We have had no complaints from patients about reduction of breast sensation, although we have not performed any special tests on sensitivity.

Skin Excess

The most frequent complication is excess skin on the inferior pole of the breast, which occurs in approximately 10% of cases. It can be caused by two factors: (1) A too high positioning of the pedicle, producing a dead space in the inferior pole and consequently an area of skin excess; and (2) an insufficient excision of skin in the inferior end of the vertical incision. It is absolutely essential to be on the lookout during the operation for the presence of a dog ear at this point. Revision is accomplished through a vertical excision that should not extend beyond the submammary sulcus. If such a maneuver cannot be performed, a T-shaped outline is made to permit the correction without adversely risking the aesthetic result.

Positioning of the Areola

The second most frequent complication is improper positioning of the nipple-areola complex in 6% of cases. To correct an anomalous position of the areola, a secondary procedure is required. Point A is marked in its correct position, and a wedge resection of the skin is performed in the upper area. Dermal stitches with inverted knots anchor the incision. Immobilization, as after the original procedure, is indispensable after a revision.

Scars

Enlargement of the vertical and/or areolar scar is present in 5% of patients. We believe this is due to technical reasons, either because of improper closure or because of inadequate compensation for the excess skin around the areola. The solution is simple: revi-

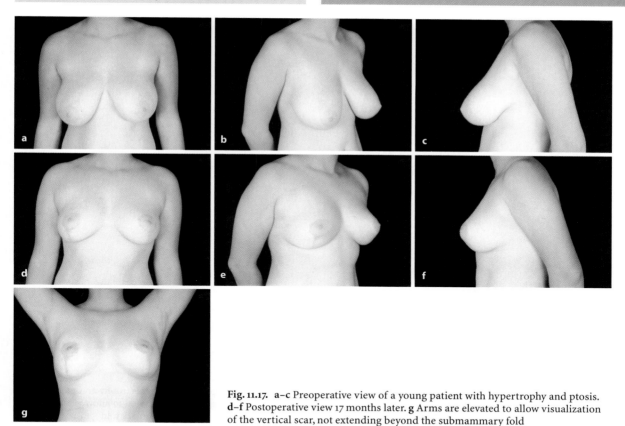

Fig. 11.17. a–c Preoperative view of a young patient with hypertrophy and ptosis. **d–f** Postoperative view 17 months later. **g** Arms are elevated to allow visualization of the vertical scar, not extending beyond the submammary fold

sion of the scars with new anchoring of the skin and immobilization. If scar hypertrophy or keloid occurs, radiation therapy is advised. No revision should be undertaken until at least 6 months after the original operation. This is the time required for the skin to retract, for the inflammatory reaction to subside, and for a more definitive shape of the operated breast to emerge.

Discussion

In mammaplasty achieving an aesthetic shape with the shortest scar possible and longest-lasting results has been the aim of most plastic surgeons. However, no single technique can accomplish all these goals. A great variety of surgical techniques are available. Vertical scar mammaplasty has allowed a significant reduction of scar length by eliminating the horizontal scar, with less resection of skin. As most vertical scar mammaplasties rely on the support of the skin envelope, a greater incidence of recurrent ptosis of the breast and healing problems in the vertical scar, such as wound dehiscence, is expected. To prevent these problems, some authors use additional measures that include fixation of the remaining gland to the pectoralis fascia with several sutures [10, 11], dermal suspension techniques [4], and even alloplastic mesh [5].

The lozenge technique is based on the skin markings of Arié [1], Peixoto's concept of tissue retraction [13, 14], and the inferiorly based pedicle. The major component of this technique and the main difference from the other techniques is the use of the inferiorly based flap called the inferior pedicle that provides good suspension for the breast as it is fixed on the pectoralis muscle and fascia, reducing the effect of gravitational pull, with better and longer-lasting results. It also provides bulk and natural fullness superiorly and inferiorly (Figs. 11.17, 11.18). Another point of concern is avoiding the extension of the vertical scar beyond the submammary sulcus. This is done by marking point D 3.0 cm above the sulcus.

Although we have had no complaints about loss of breast sensation, especially of the nipple-areola complex, a decrease in the vibration and temperature sensibility of the nipple-areola complex, particularly after large reductions, is expected [6]. It is important to keep an eye out during the surgery for the presence of a dog ear in the inferior pole of the breast, especially at the inferior end of the vertical scar, to avoid the

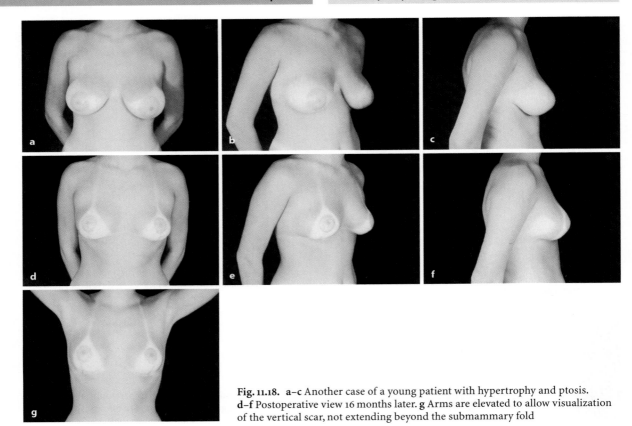

Fig. 11.18. a–c Another case of a young patient with hypertrophy and ptosis.
d–f Postoperative view 16 months later. **g** Arms are elevated to allow visualization
of the vertical scar, not extending beyond the submammary fold

need for secondary revision. The technique has proved safe with respect to viability of the tissues, especially the nipple-areola complex and the inferior pedicle.

Conclusion

The use of the inferior pedicle, in association with the principles of skin retraction, has led to the development of the lozenge technique. Prior to the operation patients must understand that a revision is possible and that the end result takes several months. The single vertical scar is an advantage and can be achieved only if patience is practiced by both patient and surgeon. Despite our satisfaction with the lozenge technique, we are certain that there will be subsequent improvements. We offer this technique as a contribution to reduction mammaplasty today and possibly a bridge to better procedures in the future.

References

1. Arié G (1957) Nueva técnica em mamaplastia. Rev Latino Am Cir Plast 3:23
2. Berthe JV, Massaut J, Greuse M, Coessens B, DeMey A (2003) The vertical mammaplasty: a reappraisal of the technique and its complications. Plast Reconstr Surg 111:2192
3. Dartigues L (1925) Traitement chirurgical du prolapsus mammaire. Arch Franco-Belg Chir 28:313
4. Exner K, Scheufler O (2002) Dermal suspension flap in vertical-scar reduction mammaplasty. Plast Reconstr Surg 109:2289
5. Góes JCS (2002) Periareolar mammaplasty: double-skin technique with application of mesh support. Clin Plastic Surg 29:349
6. Greuse M, Hamdi M, DeMey A (2001) Breast sensitivity after vertical mammaplasty. Plast Reconstr Surg 107:970
7. Hammond DC (1999) Short scar periareolar inferior pedicle reduction (SPAIR) mammaplasty. Plast Reconstr Surg 103:890
8. Joseph J (1931) Nasenplastik und sonstige gesichtplastik nebst einen ahnag ueber mammaplastik. Curt Kabitzsch, Leipzig
9. Juri J, Jari C, Cutini J, Colagno A (1982) Vertical mammaplasty. Ann Plast Surg 9:298
10. Lassus C (1996) A 30-year experience with vertical mammaplasty. Plast Reconstr Surg 97:373

11. Lejour M (1994) Vertical mammaplasty and liposuction of the breast. Plast Reconstr Surg 94:100
12. Lotsch F (1923) Über Hangebrustplastik. Zentralbl Chir 50:1241
13. Peixoto G (1980) Reduction mammaplasty: a personal technique. Plast Reconstr Surg 65:217
14. Peixoto G (1990) Reduction mammaplasty: a personal view. In: Goldwyn RM (ed) Reduction Mammaplasty. Little, Brown, Boston, p 337
15. Pitanguy I (1960) Breast hypertrophy. In: Transactions of the International Society of Plastic Surgeons, London, 1959. Livingstone, Edinburgh, p 509

16. Ribeiro L, Baker E (1973) Mastoplastia con pedículo de seguridad. Rer Esp Cir Plast 16:223
17. Ribeiro L (1989) Cirurgia plástica da mama. Medsi, Rio de Janeiro
18. Ribeiro L (1990) The lozenge technique. In: Goldwyn RM (ed) Reduction Mammaplasty. Little, Brown, Boston, p 365
19. Skoog T (1963) A technique of breast reduction. Acta Chir Scand 126:453
20. Strombeck JO (1961) Mammaplasty: report of a new technique based on the two-pedicle procedure. Br J Plast Surg 13:79

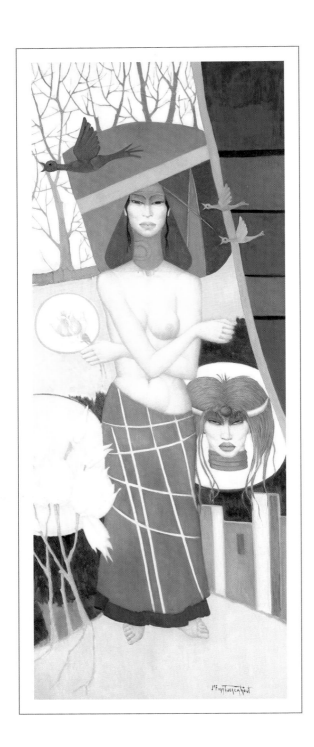

12

The Use of Vertical Scar Techniques in Reconstructive Surgery

Moustapha Hamdi, Phillip Blondeel, Koenraad Van Landuyt, Stan Monstrey

He who does not possess a thing cannot give it.

Folk tradition

Introduction

The loss of a breast or part of it can be a major impairment to a woman's body image and feeling of attractiveness. Therefore, reconstructive surgery has developed techniques that provide good aesthetic results. The plastic surgeon, who is involved in breast reconstruction after breast cancer, should have a comprehensive understanding of the biology, natural history, risk factors, and treatment of breast cancer. Psychological factors associated with cancer compound those that come into play following any body deformity, and these must be taken into account by the surgeon. In addition, actual breast reconstruction requires a working knowledge of the full range of aesthetic surgical procedures of the breast as well as the spectrum of breast reconstruction techniques. The ultimate goal of the reconstructive procedure is to achieve good aesthetic, long-lasting results with adequate symmetry.

General Considerations

Many factors should be considered in planning breast reconstruction:
- Stage of the disease: tumor size, palpable lymph nodes.
- type of ablative surgery:
  - Conservative treatment: tumorectomy or quadrantectomy.
  - Mastectomy: modified radical versus skin sparing versus subcutaneous mastectomy.
- Therapy: chemotherapy, irradiation.
- General risk factors: smoking, diabetes, etc.
- Patient expectation.

Depending on the timing of the reconstruction, whether primary or secondary, specific points should be investigated and discussed with the patient:
- Scar position.
- Nipple-areola preservation.
- Size of the reconstructed breast.
- History of previous irradiation.
- Status of contralateral breast: indications for prophylactic mastectomy, mastopexy, reduction or augmentation, or no surgery.

Vertical Scar in Reconstructive Procedures

Clinical applications of vertical scar techniques in reconstructive procedure can be divided into four categories:

Mastectomy Through a Vertical Incision

The standard modified radical mastectomy includes removal of the breast gland with the nipple-areola complex (NAC) as well as the skin overlying the tumor. However, more conservative techniques have been used if the tumor is not too close to the skin. Periareolar incision is used widely nowadays to perform the mastectomy, which allows the removal of the gland with the NAC. Besides immediate reconstruction, excellent aesthetic results can be obtained. A vertical component can be added to the periareolar incision in the following cases:
- If the NAC is small, which does not allow for gland removal.
- Reducing the size of the skin pocket to achieve a smaller size of the reconstructed breast.
- Removal of the skin over the tumor using elliptic skin excision as part of a vertical scar mammaplasty.

In the first case, we prefer to increase the access to the breast by a vertical incision because this scar usually heals well with good quality. Moreover, a mastopexy can be carried out better through this scar should the patient need a further correction in the future.

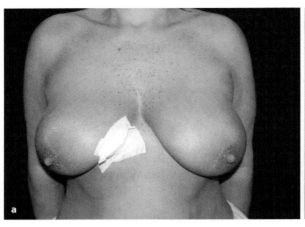
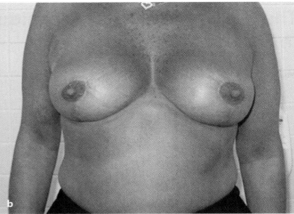

Fig. 12.1. a Preoperative view: patient who had a breast cancer located at the inferomedial quadrant as marked by *harpoon*. **b** Postoperative view: the breast was remodeled by a vertical scar mammaplsty with a superior pedicle after tumor resection

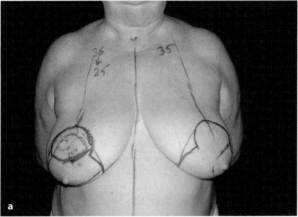
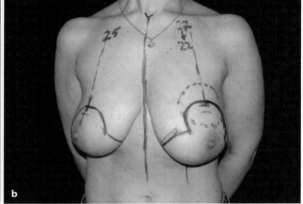

Fig. 12.2. a A patient who had a breast cancer above the nipple-areola complex but within the incision lines. The pedicle can be designed either laterally or medially to fill the defect post quad-rantectomy. **b** A patient with a tumor located above the nipple-areola complex and extended beyond the incision lines

In the last two cases, the design of vertical scar mammaplasty can be done to immediately reduce the reconstructed breast or to fit the incision pattern in such a way that the skin overlying the tumor is included within the vertical mammaplasty either within the dome-shaped excision around the NAC or within the vertical elliptic excision.

Oncoplastic Surgery

Oncologically, breast-conserving surgery for cancer, associated with postoperative radiotherapy, has proved safe as compared with total mastectomy for tumors up to 3 cm in diameter. Larger tumors are still treated with mastectomy as the first choice. However,

more efficient protocols of neoadjuvant chemotherapy may allow a more conservative local approach to advanced tumors. The combination of a quardantectomy with an immediate partial breast reconstruction is considered a decisive stage in the evolution of breast cancer surgery. This combination, so-called "oncoplastic surgery," allows a wider resection of the tumor with safe margins, together with the advantages of the immediate breast reconstruction by using a supple, malleable nonirradiated tissue in order to achieve both ultimate goals: adequate local control of the disease and good aesthetic results (Fig. 12.1a, b).

Here, too, a vertical mammaplasty pattern can be designed to incorporate the tumor excision within the lines of incision (Fig. 12.2a). The pattern can be rotated laterally or medially to fit the location of the tumor.

Table 12.1. Choice of pedicle depending on location of defect

Location of defect	Vertical scar mammaplasty
Inferior, inferomedial, or inferolateral	Superior, superomedial, or superolateral pedicle
Superior	Inferior or centroinferior pedicle
Superomedial	Superolateral pedicle with an inferocentral component to fill the defect
Superolateral	Superomedial pedicle with an inferocentral component to fill the defect
Central	Inferior pedicle (Grisotti's flap)

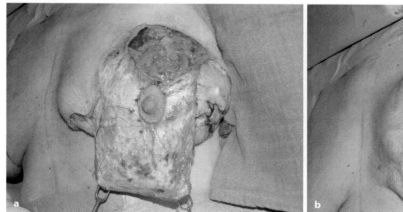
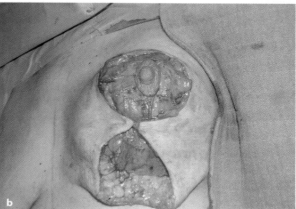

Fig. 12.3 a,b. Preoperative views of the same patient in Fig. 12.2b. **a** A centroinferior pedicle was designed to reconstruct the defect. **b** The pedicle was transferred and fixed cranially to the pectoralis fascia and the skin

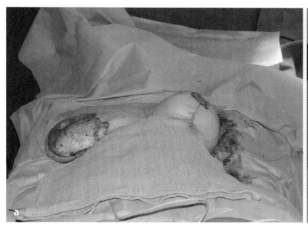
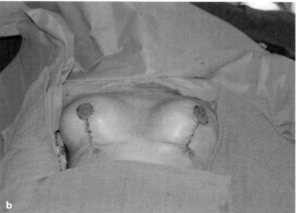

Fig. 12.4. a The remodeled breast was closed with a vertical scar technique. **b** A contralateral breast was remodeled by a vertical scar mammaplasty with a superior pedicle to achieve better symmetry

If the tumor crosses over the incision line, a suitable pedicle should be designed to reconstruct the defect (Fig. 12.2 b). The choice of the pedicle is related to tumor location (Table 12.1). Good knowledge of the breast blood supply is essential for designing different potential pedicles to carry the NAC or to reconstruct the defect. Depending on the tumor's location, different pedicles can be selected (Figs. 12.3, 12.4).

The reconstructed breast should be made 10% larger than the contralateral remodeled breast be-

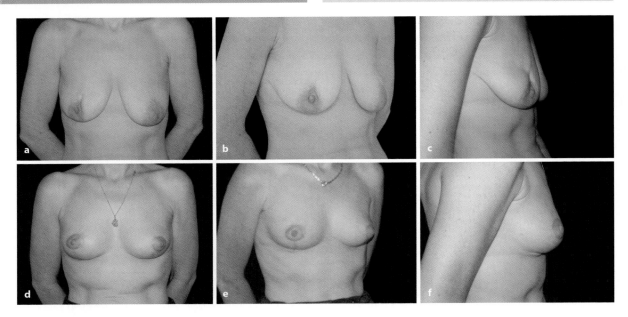

Fig. 12.5. a–c Preoperative views: a patient who had a conserving right breast therapy left with retroareolar defect. **d–f** Postoperative views: the results after vertical scar mastopexy with a superior pedicle

cause one should expect some shrinking and changing in the volume of the reconstructed breast due to the irradiation. Some of the relative anatomical contraindications for oncoplastic surgery are large tumor/breast ratio and tumor location behind the nipple. However, the use of local or distant flaps can provide additional tissue in specific cases.

Correction of Breast Deformity after Conservative Therapy

The same application of an immediate partial breast reconstruction may be used in the case of a breast deformity after conservative therapy. However, more care must be taken in using surgical techniques of mammaplasty. These cases are usually more challenging because of the irradiation's effect on the breast tissue, which leads to much less malleable and poorly vascularized tissues. The same algorithm described above in pedicle choosing can still be used (Fig. 12.5).

Nevertheless, techniques in mammaplasty should be adapted to this specific situation. A minimal skin undermining with a short and wide pedicle must be used. Experience has shown that a high rate of complications and less aesthetic results are obtained in a secondary correction compared to the immediate partial breast reconstruction. Wound dehiscence, fat necrosis, and infection are more expected in irradiated tissues, and patients who require breast correction should be aware of the potential higher risks of complications. In addition, a defect on the superoexternal

location may lead to a major nipple-areola displacement. The combination of a large amount of scar tissue due both to tumorectomy and axillary lymph node dissection and to irradiation makes the defect too difficult to correct by mammaplasty techniques alone. In this specific case, a locoregional tissue transfer is required. Pedicled flaps from the axillary region may still be available, but pedicled latissimus dorsi, scapular, or perforator flaps might be better options for resolving this problem.

Remodeling the Contralateral Breast

Patients who undergo a breast reconstructive procedure may require surgery of the contralateral breast in order to obtain a better breast symmetry or to improve the aesthetic appearance of both breasts. First, the reconstructed breast should be shaped higher and smaller in accordance with the patient's wishes. Corrections of the contralateral breast are rarely performed together with breast reconstruction, for two reasons: the reconstructed breast will undergo changes in shape after sagging, absorption of edema, and hematoma postoperatively; or the reconstructed breast will change as a result of possible irradiation. It is advisable to delay the correction of the contralateral breast to a second stage within 3 to 6 months. Immediate remodeling is usually done in cases of oncoplastic surgery in which a bilateral remodeling of both breasts is performed as part of the surgical procedure.

References

1. Simmons RM, Fish SK, Gayle L, La Trenta GS, Swistel A, Christos P, Osborne MP (1999) Local and distant recurrence rates in skin-sparing mastectomies compared with non-skin-sparing mastectomies. Ann Surg Oncol 6:676

2. Rowland JH (1998) Psychological impact of treatments for breast cancer. In: Spear SL (ed) Surgery of the Breast. Lippi-cott-Raven, Philadelphia, p 295

3. Sufi PA, Gittos M, Collier DS (2000) Envelope mastectomy with immediate reconstruction (EMIR). Eur J Surg Oncol 26:367

4. Hidalgo DA, Borgen PJ, Petrek JA, Heerdt AH, Cody HS, Disa JJ (1998) Immediate reconstruction after complete skin-sparing mastectomy with autologous tissue. J Am Coll Surg 187:17

5. Hammond DC, Capraro PA, Ozolins EB, Arnold JF (2002) Use of a skin-sparing reduction pattern to create a combination skin-muscle flap pocket in immediate breast reconstruction. Plast Reconstr Surg 110:206

6. Disa JJ, Cordeiro PG, Heerdt AH, Petrek JA, Borgen PJ, Hidalgo DA (2003) Skin-sparing mastectomy and immediate autologous tissue reconstruction after whole-breast irradiation. Plast Reconstr Surg 111:118

7. Spear SL, Pelletiere CV, Wolfe AJ, Tsangaris TN, Pennanen MF (2003) Experience with reduction mammaplasty combined with breast conservation therapy in the treatment of breast cancer. Plast Reconstr Surg 111:1102

8. Veronesi U, Cascinelli N, Mariani L, Greco M, Saccozzi R, Luini A, Aguilar M, Marubini E (2002). Twenty-year follow-up of a randomized study comparing breast-conserving surgery with radical mastectomy for early breast cancer. N Engl J Med 347:1227

9. Fisher B, Anderson S, Bryant J, Margolese RG, Deutsch M, Fisher ER, Jeong JH, Wolmark N (2002) Twenty-year follow-up of a randomized trial comparing total mastectomy, lumpectomy, and lumpectomy plus irradiation for the treatment of invasive breast cancer. N Engl J Med 347: 1233

10. Salvin SA, Love SM, Padousky NL (1992) Reconstruction of the radiated partial mastectomy defect with autogenous tissue. Plast Reconstr Surg 90:854

11. Losken A, Carlson GW, Bostwick J III, Jones GE, Culbertson JH, Schoemann M (2002) Trends in unilateral breast reconstruction and management of the contralateral breast: the Emory experience. Plast Reconstr Surg 110:89

12. Malata CM, Hodgson EL, Chikwe J, Canal AC, Purushotham AD (2003) An application of the LeJour vertical mammaplasty pattern for skin-sparing mastectomy: a preliminary report. Ann Plast Surg 51:345

13. Petit JY, Garusi C, Greuse M, Rietiens M, Youssef O, Luini A, De Lorenzi F (2002) One hundred and eleven cases of breast conservation treatment with simultaneous reconstruction at the European Institute of Oncology (Milan). Tumori 88:41

14. Grisotti A (1994) Immediate reconstruction after partial mastectomy. Oper Tech Plast Reconstr Surg 1:1

15. Clough KB, Cuminet J, Fitoussi A, Nos C, Mosseri V (1998) Cosmetic sequelae after conservative treatment for breast cancer: classification and results of surgical correction. Ann Plast Surg 41:471

16. Clough KB, Kroll SS, Audretsch W (1999) An approach to the repair of partial mastectomy defects. Plast Reconstr Surg 104:409

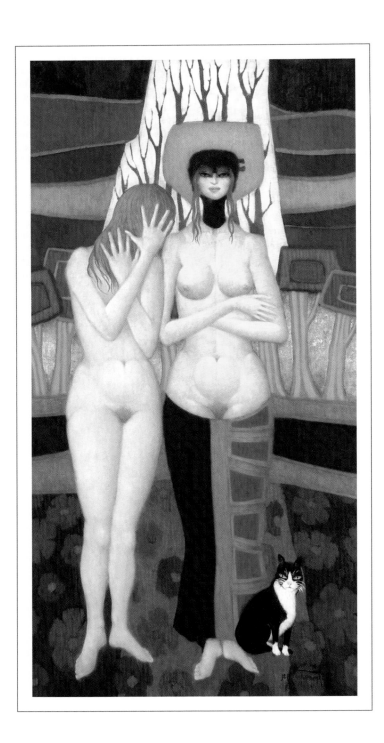

Vertical Reduction and Mastopexy: Problems and Solutions

M. Keith Hanna, Foad Nahai

13

It does a bullet no good to go fast; and a man,
if he be truly a man, no harm to go slow; for
his glory is not at all in going, but in being.

John Ruskin

Introduction

To a certain extent all surgical techniques evolve over time as a consequence of attempts to improve results and prevent complications. The same can be said of the evolution of vertical mammaplasty. The early goals of breast reduction revolved around the search for a reliable technique to transpose the nipple-areola complex. The 1960s saw the introduction of the superior pedicle by Arie [1] and Pitanguy [2], as well as the horizontal bipedicle by Strombeck [3] and the lateral cutaneous pedicle by Skoog [4]. The vertical bipedicle method was popularized by McKissock [5, 6] in the 1970s. During the 1980s and 1990s the inferior pedicle [7–10] became the technique of choice for surgeons in North America due to its ease and reliability. Concurrent with the evolution of reliable pedicles for nipple-areola transposition was the implementation of the Wise pattern skin markings, which resulted in an inverted T-shaped scar. The unsightly appearance of the horizontal inframammary scar in some patients spurred the next step in the evolution of breast reduction techniques, the vertical scar mammaplasty.

In 1970, Lassus [11] described a vertical scar breast reduction technique with a superior pedicle. The problem with the initial technique was that the vertical scars were often below the inframammary fold. This problem was addressed by Marchac and de Olarte [12] through the addition of a short horizontal inframammary scar. Lejour [13–16] then popularized the vertical breast reduction in the 1990s. She combined gland suturing to the pectoralis fascia, to preserve breast shape, with extensive skin undermining, especially inferiorly with gathering of the vertical scar, to maintain the scar above the inframammary crease. She also utilized extensive liposuction for

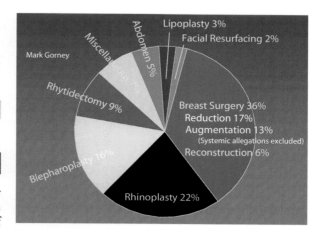

Fig. 13.1. Malpractice claims filed from Corney [28]

breast contouring. This technique was applied by many surgeons for small reductions but was not as well received for large reductions due to the increased incidence of vertical scar healing problems [17, 18]. In the last few years many modifications have been proposed in an attempt to reduce complications and to make this technique more applicable to larger breast reductions [17–21]. Basically these modifications included elimination of gland suturing to the chest wall, fewer internal gland sutures, minimizing skin undermining, and avoiding liposuction or limiting it to the lateral breast and axillary areas.

No operations are without problems or complications, and breast reduction is no exception. Looking at aesthetic surgery as a whole, breast reduction surgery in the U.S. is second only to rhinoplasty in the number of malpractice claims filed over the last 10 years (Fig. 13.1). Most problems are common to all breast reduction techniques and involve nipple-areola viability, nipple-areola sensation, delayed healing, scars, breast shape and projection, nipple malposition, hematoma, seroma, and infection (Table 13.1). The most serious complication is nipple-areola/breast necrosis, while the most common problem is imperfection of breast shape. The incidence of complications and revision rates associated with limited incision breast surgery are related to the learning curve, body mass index (BMI), breast size, and skin manage-

Table 13.1 Problems common to all breast reduction techniques

Immediate problems	Delayed problems
Nipple-areola viability	Delayed healing
Hematoma	Scars
Seroma	Breast shape and projection
Infection	Nipple malposition

Table 13.2. Factors related to the incidence of complications and revision rates in limited incision breast surgery

Learning curve
Body mass index (BMI)
Breast size
Skin management

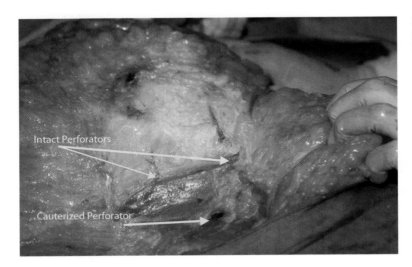

Fig. 13.2. Intact perforators to superior pedicle, cauterized perforator to central and inferior pedicle

ment (Table 13.2). It is our experience and opinion, as well as of others [15, 22], that the rate and severity of complications are related more to patient BMI and breast size than to the type of operation performed. In this chapter we will discuss the problems associated with vertical scar mammaplasty and possible preventative solutions.

Complications: General Considerations

Immediate Problems

Nipple-Areola Viability

No pedicle is without risk regardless of technique used. We have all seen nipple-areola problems with all types of pedicles. While the superior pedicle used with vertical reduction is reliable, the dermal extension may not always be as dependable. Breast size or volume of resection is not as important to nipple viability as the distance upwards that the nipple has to move.

To reduce complications with nipple-areola viability, a number of possible preemptive measures should be considered. The surgeon should always be diligent to recognize and preserve perforators to the superior pedicle in order to avoid injury to the arterial supply of the nipple-areola complex (Fig. 13.2). Therefore, a thorough understanding of the arterial anatomy of the breast is essential for avoiding tissue loss. Another caveat is that the longer the pedicle, the thinner it should be in order to facilitate insetting of the areola (Fig. 13.3). It is important to bear in mind also that the longer the pedicle, the wider it must be in order to preserve vascularity (Fig. 13.4). If difficulty is encountered with insetting the areola, cautious liposuction can be used to make this possible. In high-risk patients, a double pedicle (i.e., vertical bipedicle) should be considered.

Blue discoloration of the areola after insetting is a sign of venous impairment and is usually due to either tension on the areola or kinking of the pedicle. This change in color is a sign of impending necrosis and should be addressed immediately. If signs of venous compression are present, the sutures should be removed and the cause of the tension or twisting corrected (Fig. 13.5).

Fig. 13.8. Nipple position too high, right breast

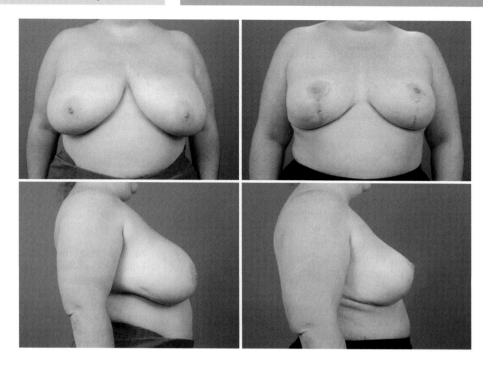

Table 13.4. Statistical reviews of complications with different breast reduction techniques

Author	Technique	Seroma	Hematoma	Infection	Partial areola loss	Delayed wound healing	Revision rate
[15]	Lejour	4.2%	1%		1%	4.2%	
[16]	Lejour	5%	1.3%	0.4%	0.4%	5.5%	
[27]	Lejour					40%	20%
[17]	Lejour	16%	5%	9%		18%	16%
[18]	Lejour					6%	7%
Author	**Technique**	**Minor complication**				**Major complication**	**Revision rate**
[21]	Lejour	30%			15%	28%	
	Modified Lejour	15%			5%	22%	
Author	**Technique**	**Total complications**				**Delayed wound healing**	
[24]	Wise	53%	19%			19%	
[26]	Wise	20%					
[25]	Wise	41%	29%			29%	

showed a 41% complication rate and 29% delayed healing. Obviously, complications and delayed healing are observed in all methods of breast reduction (Table 13.4).

Conclusion

The technique of vertical reduction mammaplasty continues to evolve as we endeavor to improve results and prevent complications. The technique as described by Lassus and popularized by Lejour is not trouble free. However, the incidence of complications is no higher than that of Wise pattern procedures. These complications can be minimized through an understanding of the underlying causes, familiarity with the technique, and patient selection.

References

1. Arie G (1957) Una nueva tecnica de mastoplastia. Rev Iber Latinoam Cir Plast 3:28
2. Pitanguy I (1967) Surgical correction of breast hypertrophy. Br J Plast Surg 20:78
3. Strombeck JO (1960) Mammaplasty: report of a new technique based on the two-pedicle procedure. Br J Plast Surg 13:79
4. Skoog T (1963) A technique of breast reduction – transposition of the nipple on a cutaneous vascular pedicle. Acta Chir Scand 126:453
5. McKissock PK (1972) Reduction mammaplasty with a vertical dermal flap. Plast Reconstr Surg 49:245
6. McKissock PK (1976) Reduction mammaplasty by the vertical bipedicle flap technique: rationale and results. Clin Plast Surg 3:309
7. Ribeiro L (1975) A new technique for reduction mammaplasty. Plast Reconstr Surg 55:330
8. Robbins TH (1997) A reduction mammaplasty with the areola-nipple based on an inferior pedicle. Plast Reconstr Surg 59:64
9. Courtiss EH, Goldwyn RM (1997) Reduction mammaplasty by the inferior pedicle technique: an alternative to free nipple and areola grafting for severe macromastia or extreme ptosis. Plast Reconstr Surg 59:500
10. Georgiade NG, Serafin D, Morris R, Georgiade G (1979) Reduction mammaplasty utilizing an inferior pedicle nipple-areolar flap. Ann Plast Surg 3:211
11. Lassus C (1970) A technique for breast reduction. Int Surg 53:69
12. Marchac D, de Olarte G (1982) Reduction mammaplasty and correction of ptosis with a short inframammary scar. Plast Reconstr Surg 69:45
13. Lejour M, Abboud M (1990) Vertical mammaplasty without inframammary scar and with breast liposuction. Perspect Plast Surg 4:67
14. Lejour M, Abboud M, Declety A, Kertesz P (1990) Réduction des cicatrices de plastie mammaire: de l'ancre courte à la verticale. Ann Chir Plast Esthet 35:369
15. Lejour M (1994) Vertical Mammaplasty and Liposuction of the Breast. Quality Medical Publishing, St Louis
16. Lejour M (1994) Vertical mammaplasty and liposuction of the breast. Plast Reconstr Surg 94:100
17. Leone MS, Franchelli S, Berrino P, Santi PL (1997) Vertical mammaplasty: a personal approach. Aesthetic Plast Surg 21:356
18. Palumbo SK, Shifren J, Rhee C (1998) Modifications of the Lejour vertical mammaplasty: analysis of results in 100 consecutive patients. Ann Plast Surg 40:354
19. Hall-Findlay EJ (1999) A simplified vertical reduction mammaplasty: shortening the learning curve. Plast Reconstr Surg 104:748
20. Beer GM, Morgenthaler W, Spicher I, Meyer VE (2001) Modifications in vertical scar breast reduction. Br J Plast Surg 54:341
21. Berthe J, Massaut J, Greuse M, Coessens B, De May A (2003) The vertical mammaplasty: a reappraisal of the technique and its complications. Plast Reconstr Surg 111:2192
22. Lejour M (1999) Vertical mammaplasty: early complications after 250 personal consecutive cases. Plast Reconstr Surg 104:764
23. McKissock PK (1984) Complications and undesirable results with reduction mammaplasty. In: Goldwyn RM (ed) The Unfavorable Result in Plastic Surgery: Avoidance and Treatment, 2nd edn. Little, Brown, Boston, pp 739
24. Davis GM, Ringler SL, Short K, Serrick D, Bengston BP (1995) Reduction mammaplasty: long-term efficacy, morbidity, and patient satisfaction. Plast Reconstr Surg 96:1106
25. Makki AS, Ghanem AA (1998) Long-term results and patient satisfaction with reduction mammaplasty. Ann Plast Surg 41:370
26. Schnur PL, Schnur DP, Petty PM, Hanson TJ, Weaver AL (1997) Reduction mammaplasty: an outcome study. Plast Reconstr Surg 100:875
27. Pickford MA, Boorman JG (1993) Early experience with the Lejour vertical scar reduction mammaplasty technique. Br J Plast Surg 46:516
28. Gorney M (2000) Ten years' experience in aesthetic surgery malpractice claims. Aesthetic Plast Surg 21:569

14

Secondary Revisions after Vertical Scar Mammaplasty

Moustapha Hamdi

> I never doubted a truth that needed an explanation unless I found myself having to analyse the explanation.
>
> *Khalil Gibran*

Introduction

Vertical scar or reduced scar mammaplasty has been a major advance in breast reduction techniques. The aim of the techniques is to obtain an excellent aesthetic appearance that is long lasting but with minimal scars. Attempts to reduce the scarring in breast reduction should not however compromise the aesthetic result. This may occur, though, particularly in the early stages of any new technique.

When the contributing authors of this book were asked to provide an overview of the need for secondary revision, the response was immediate and unambiguous: "few," "rare," "seldom," "unusual," etc. This is largely due to the immense experience of the faculty who have spent years developing and optimizing their techniques.

Complications can, however, still occur, and they may necessitate revision surgery. Complication rates of up to 40% have been reported in the literature (Chap. 13). Fortunately, not all of these complications require secondary surgery – many can be solved by conservative treatment. Nevertheless, secondary revisions of various vertical scar mammaplasty techniques have been reported in 4–28% of cases. In addition, significant breast ptosis or massive breast reduction often necessitates "tidy-up" procedures. This chapter gives an overview of the secondary procedures required to correct complications or unsatisfactory results.

Revision Procedures

Revision of an unsatisfactory breast reduction procedure can be one of the most difficult breast reconstructions. As always, it is easier to operate on one's own complications because the surgeon knows which technique was previously used and what difficulties were encountered. Reviewing the preoperative and postoperative pictures may help in analysis of the problem and aid in preventing unsatisfactory results in the future. In the case of a referred patient, the surgeon requires adequate information concerning the relevant past medical history of the patient, preoperative status of the breast, surgical technique used, and postoperative course. Patients requiring further correction should be treated cautiously, and direct contact with the previous surgeon is preferable. Precise description of the perceived or actual problem, good documentation of the clinical picture, and excellent communication with the patient are vital for ensuring a well-prepared patient and avoiding any potential malpractice claims.

The need for secondary revision can be summarized in five categories.

Revisions Related to Scars

Hypertrophic or keloid scars can occur with any surgical episode, and the standard treatment protocols of pressure dressing, silicon gels, and/or local corticosteroid injections should be employed as necessary. Most scars respond to conservative treatment. Persistent reddish or dark scars can improve by pulsed ruby laser therapy. Resistant keloid scarring with significant symptoms (pain, irritation, pruritis) may occasionally require reexcision and brachytherapy (iridium threads). It is rare to see scar hypertrophy of the vertical limb after breast reduction; when it does occur, it is usually at the inferior pole of the vertical scar if it crosses the inframammary fold (IMF). In fact, the low rate of vertical scar hypertrophy is one of the major advantages of vertical scar techniques; they bypass many of the difficulties of the inverted T scar techniques.

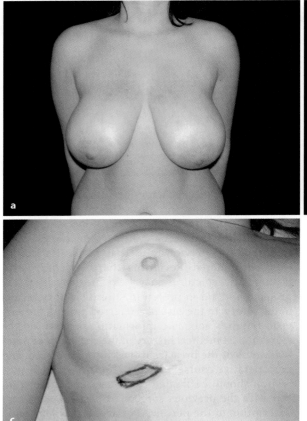
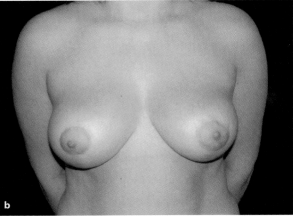

Fig. 14.1 a–c. A 29-year-old patient who had a moderate breast reduction using the septum-based lateral mammaplasty (SLM, Dr. Hamdi). a, b Preoperative and postoperative views. c Revision under local anesthesia was necessary at the base of the vertical scar

Wide or malpositioned scars more frequently occur at the base of the vertical scar. Using a pursestring suture at this level during initial surgery is a good option for shortening the vertical wound and for keeping the scar above the IMF; however, it may still result in a wide scar with persistent wrinkles. Such scars are usually easily corrected by reexcision and meticulous closure (Fig. 14.1). The vertical scar is more difficult to correct when it crosses the IMF. In this case, the scar can be elevated by a crescentic excision that incorporates the bottom of the wound into the IMF; this is in conjunction with liposuction on either side of the scar to avoid new dog ears. These simple corrections are amenable to local anesthesia. The wise surgeon should make the patient aware of the need for occasional "tidy-up" procedures at the initial consultation, especially in the case of large breasts. Taping of the scar postoperatively may reduce problems significantly. Correction is ideally performed 3 months after the initial surgery in order to allow wound healing and skin retraction to take place.

Revisions Related to Skin Excess

Persistent skin excess, usually the most frequent complication, occurs at the inferior pole of the breast and is reported in approximately 10 % of cases of vertical scar mammaplasty. It may be caused by various factors:

1. Excessively high positioning of the pedicle, producing a dead space in the inferior pole and subsequent skin excess.
2. Insufficient excision of skin at the inferior end of the vertical incision (Figs. 14.2, 14.3). It is absolutely essential to look for potential dog ears at this point during surgery and to correct them immediately.
3. In larger reductions of more than 1000 g, postoperative resolution of swelling can sometimes result in a lax skin envelope in the lower pole. Simple excision of the redundant skin along the previous vertical incision reshapes the lower pole of the breast and restores a pleasing contour without additional scarring. Also, tightening of the lower skin enve-

Fig. 14.2 a–d. A middle-aged patient with breast hypertrophy and marked ptosis who had reduction of 300 g on the right and 330 g on the left breast using the inferocentral pedicle technique (Dr. Wueringer).
a, b Preoperative and postoperative views. **c** Bilateral dog ears at the level of the IMF, which are noticeable when the patient raises her arms. **d** Marking of a crescent excision

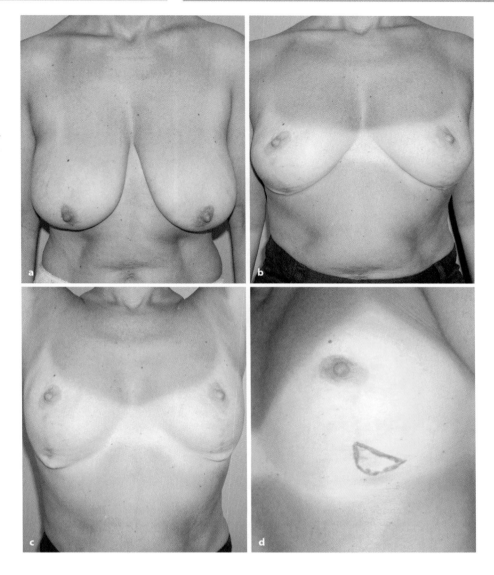

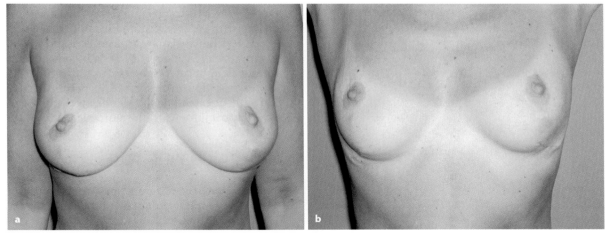

Fig. 14.3 a,b. Immediate postoperative results after the secondary revision of the scar

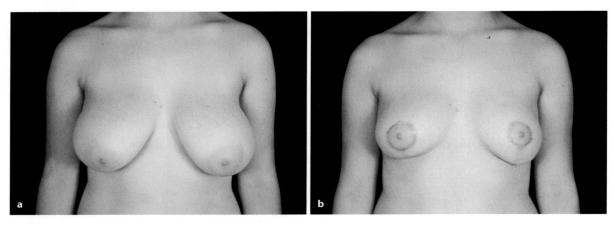

Fig. 14.4. a Preoperative view of a patient with large and ptotic breasts. **b** The patient underwent breast reduction using the lozenge technique (Dr. Ribeiro); a postoperative view demonstrates the excess of skin at the inferior pole of the left breast

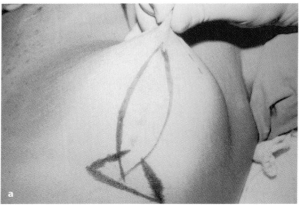 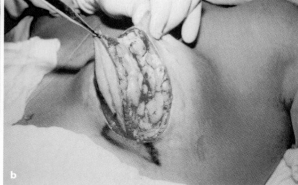

Fig. 14.5. a The area of skin resection is marked in the form of an ellipse not extending beyond the inframammary sulcus. An inverted T-shaped marking is designed in case extra skin resection is needed. **b** In this case only the vertical excision was per-

formed, including skin, fat, and glandular tissue. The final result was a vertical scar not extending beyond the inframammary fold

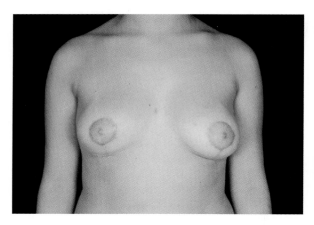

Fig. 14.6. Result after correction

lope increases the projection of the breast and often improves the overall aesthetic result. When necessary, additional tissue can also be removed via this approach (Fig. 14.4–14.6). If such a maneuver is not sufficient to correct the excess, a short T- or L-shaped resection is performed to permit correction without extending the scar below the IMF and adversely compromising the aesthetic result.

Revisions Related to Breast Shape

Unsatisfactory aesthetic results may be the result of final breast asymmetry; this may be due to insufficient gland resection on one side or to different closure methods where one breast envelope is tightened more than the other. Usually this happens if separate

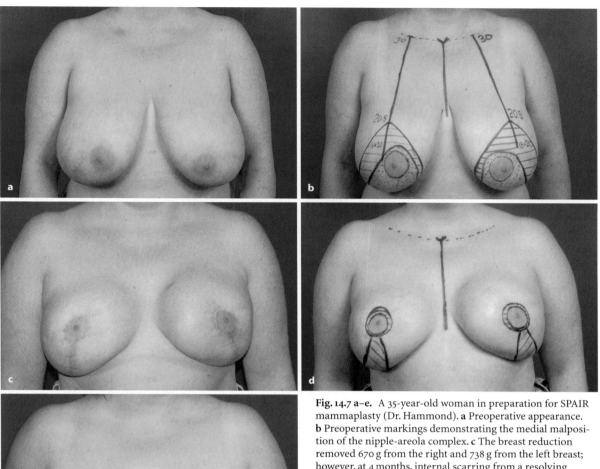

Fig. 14.7 a–e. A 35-year-old woman in preparation for SPAIR mammaplasty (Dr. Hammond). **a** Preoperative appearance. **b** Preoperative markings demonstrating the medial malposition of the nipple-areola complex. **c** The breast reduction removed 670 g from the right and 738 g from the left breast; however, at 4 months, internal scarring from a resolving bilateral seroma cavity has tethered the breast flaps and pedicle, causing shape distortion and asymmetry. **d** Preoperative marks outline the planned periareolar scar revision along with further plication of the vertical skin segment. Additional reduction of 241 g on the right and 186 g on the left breast is performed. The scarred seroma cavity is removed, restoring a pleasing shape to the breast. **e** The final result seen at 2 months after the correction shows correction of the shape distortion along with a better overall aesthetic appearance

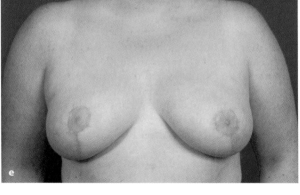

surgeons are working on each breast with little communication or if many sutures were used to shape the breast gland. We do not therefore advise the use of many fixation stitches either on the thoracic wall or between the breast pillars. Closure of the two vertical pillars is performed with stitches in the superficial fascia followed by a second layer in the dermis. Few or no stitches on the gland are recommended in order to avoid fat necrosis, which may contribute to breast asymmetry later on. Another reason for breast asymmetry is internal scarring due to seroma or hematoma formation deep within the breast. As the seroma resolves, the scar cavity that has developed pulls on the pedicle, flattening of the breast mound. If this shape distortion does not resolve satisfactorily after 1 year, it is necessary to surgically excise the scarred cavity through the previous periareolar and vertical incisions (Fig. 14.7). After removal of the scar cavity, the breast shape is restored. No instances of recurrence have been reported.

Revisions Related to Lateral Fullness

Patients with a high body mass index are at risk for developing this complication. Lateral fullness occurs more often in techniques in which a superolateral, lateral, or inferolateral pedicle is used. The fear of jeop-

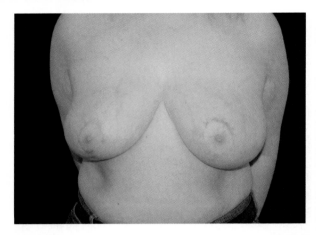

Fig. 14.8. A 28-year-old patient who underwent a breast reduction of 550 g on the right and 480 g on the left breast using the septum-based lateral mammaplasty (Dr. Hamdi). A lateral fullness is seen because of insufficient resection on the lateral side of the left breast and secondary sagging. Further excision of the skin and gland at the lateral vertical pillar is adequate to correct the problem

ardizing the blood supply to the pedicle by over resecting in this area may result in undesired fat excess (Fig. 14.8). Secondary revisions can easily be performed under local anesthetic within 3 months of the initial surgery. Alternatively, reduction mammaplasty can be performed in conjunction with liposuction to the axillary tail; this also decreases the incidence of persistent fullness. Liposuction is usually recommended at the end of reduction surgery in order to sculpt the breast and remove excess fat in regions that cannot easily be reached through the incisions.

Revisions Related to the Nipple-Areola Complex (NAC)

The most serious complication of breast reduction surgery is nipple-areola complex (NAC) or breast necrosis. Very large breasts and/or significant breast ptosis are the main reasons for such a disastrous complication, particularly in inexperienced hands. However, partial or total necrosis of the NAC can still occur in patients with high risk factors such as smoking, diabetes, or chronic corticosteroid therapy. Free nipple techniques in breast reduction are a viable alternative option for patients with large or ptotic breasts and should be considered and discussed early. Viability of the NAC depends more on adequate venous return than arterial input, with most cases of NAC necrosis being secondary to venous congestion. Methods to avoid later venous congestion include choosing

of a suitable technique, appropriate design of the pedicle, avoidance of aggressive defatting of the pedicle especially under the NAC, suitable pedicle placement without kinking or over tight fixation, and judicious drain placement if there is a dead space behind the NAC.

If the NAC demonstrates venous insufficiency at the end of surgery, liposuction of the pedicle may provide instant relief of any tension. Should the NAC congestion persist, the surgeon is duty-bound to reopen the breast and resite the pedicle in a better position. Immediate postoperative edema and swelling may cause NAC venous congestion, too, and release of the periareolar stitches is recommended in this case. Manual massage of the NAC can help to improve the venous return but should be performed with care and propriety! Medicinal leeches are not recommended because of the increased risk of infection, which may result in total NAC necrosis. Despite all these measures, partial NAC necrosis can still occur and is often better treated conservatively. This usually produces a discolored scarred region, which can later be corrected by simple scar revision with or without tattooing.

A comprehensive approach to patient care and the potential pitfalls for the NAC, along with close communication with the patient, are essential throughout. Major or total NAC necrosis will necessitate a reconstructive procedure. Wound healing may be left to occur by secondary intention; however, surgical debridement is indicated if necrosis is accompanied by infection. Direct closure can be nicely achieved using a purse-string suture. Nipple-sharing techniques may be used in cases of large contralateral nipple. Modified star techniques for nipple reconstruction are recommended when only limited viable tissue is available. In association with tattooing, the aesthetic results are usually very acceptable.

Rearrangement of the breast skin envelope coupled with increased tension on the skin closure due to swelling or widened or hypertrophic scars may occur in the periareolar location. Purse-string closure can occasionally result in persistent wrinkling around the areola or a herniated or strangulated looking areola (Fig. 14.9). After the breast has completely settled and all the postoperative swelling has resolved, simple scar revision usually greatly improves the appearance of the NAC and can completely remove any widened or hypertrophic segments without fear of recurrence. Also, once the periareolar closure has stabilized, the tendency for the purse-string closure to form persistent pleats is very much reduced. As a result, persistent periareolar wrinkling can be eliminated with simple periareolar scar revision.

Where necessary, these revision strategies can be used in combination to correct postoperative defor-

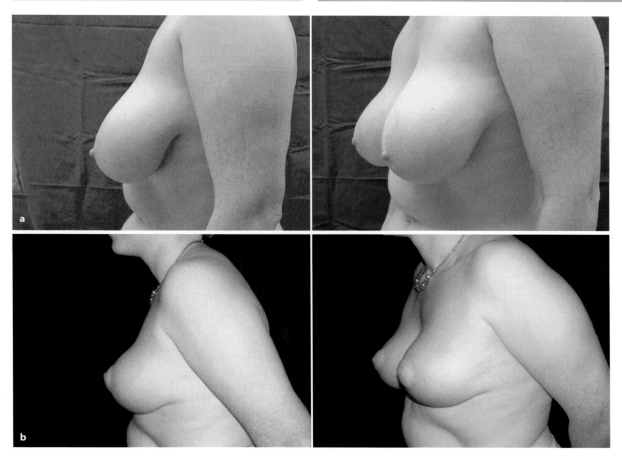

Fig. 14.9 a,b. A patient who underwent breast reduction using a septum-based medial mammaplasty (Dr. Hamdi). **a** Preoperative views. **b** Postoperative views show a nice projected but herniated looking nipple-areola complex due to the purse-string Gore-Tex stitch. A simple revision of the periareolar scar corrected this aspect without removal of the original suture

mities and to improve the overall aesthetic result. Since the combined periareolar and vertical skin resections complement one another, they are readily used in combination to correct both scars and breast shape. The access provided by these incisions allows for adequate internal reshaping as required. Taken together, these maneuvers provide straightforward solutions to complications after vertical scar mammaplasty when they do arise.

References

1. Beer GM, Morgenthaler W, Spicher I, Meyer VE (2001) Modifications in vertical scar breast reduction. Br J Plast Surg 54:341
2. Berthe J, Massaut J, Greuse M, Coessens B, De May A (2003) The vertical mammaplasty: a reappraisal of the technique and its complications. Plast Reconstr Surg 111:2192
3. Cruz-Korchin N, Korchin L (2003) Vertical versus Wise pattern breast reduction: patient satisfaction, revision rates, and complications. Plast Reconstr Surg 112:1573
4. Davis GM, Ringler SL, Short K, Serrick D, Bengston BP (1995) Reduction mammaplasty: long-term efficacy, morbidity, and patient satisfaction. Plast Reconstr Surg 96:1106
5. Hall-Findlay EJ (1999) A simplified vertical reduction mammaplasty: shortening the learning curve. Plast Reconstr Surg 104:748
6. Lassus C (1996) A 30-year experience with vertical mammaplasty. Plast Reconstr Surg 97:373
7. Lejour M (1999) Vertical mammaplasty: early complications after 250 personal consecutive cases. Plast Reconstr Surg 104:764
8. Lejour M (1999) Vertical mammaplasty: update and appraisal of late results. Plast Reconstr Surg 104:771
9. Makki AS, Ghanem AA (1998) Long-term results and patient satisfaction with reduction mammaplasty. Ann Plast Surg 41:370
10. Palumbo SK, Shifren J, Rhee C (1998) Modifications of the Lejour vertical mammaplasty: analysis of results in 100 consecutive patients. Ann Plast Surg 40:354

11. Pickford MA, Boorman JG (1993) Early experience with the Lejour vertical scar reduction mammaplasty technique. Br J Plast Surg 46:516

12. Poell MDJG (2004) Vertical reduction mammaplasty. Aesthetic Plast Surg 28(2):59

13. Rubino C, Dessay LA, Posadinu A (2003) A modified technique for nipple reconstruction: the "arrow flap". Br J Plast Surg 56:247–251

14. Schnur PL, Schnur DP, Petty PM, Hanson TJ, Weaver AL (1997) Reduction mammaplasty: an outcome study. Plast Reconstr Surg 100:875

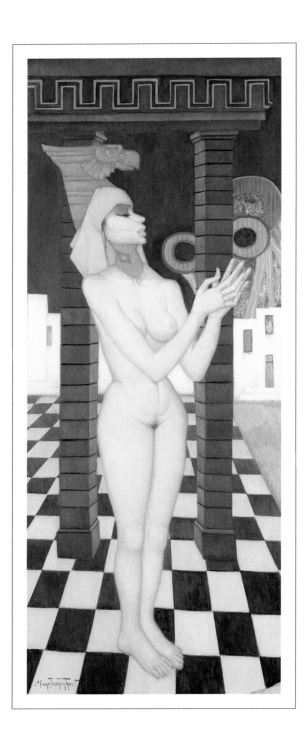

15

Indications and Contraindications of Vertical Scar Mammaplasty: General Consensus

Moustapha Hamdi

> T There are three types of people in the world. The capable person is one who can make decisions and seek advice. The half-capable person is one who can reach decisions but neglects to seek advice. The incapable person is one who can neither make decisions nor seek advice.
>
> *Folk tradition*

In this chapter I will summarize the experience of all the contributing authors and give some guidelines for young surgeons who are keen to adopt a vertical scar technique in breast reduction. All senior authors have been able to perform a vertical scar mammaplasty on every patient who had breast reduction of up to 2000 g per breast. However, in these difficult cases, only experienced surgeons are likely to obtain aesthetic results, and reductions of this magnitude are best avoided until significant experience with the technique has been obtained.

Who is the Ideal Candidate for the Vertical Mammaplasty?

In patients who have simple breast ptosis or who require only a small reduction of 400 to 500 g or less, the vertical mammaplasty can provide an excellent aesthetic result. Addition of an aggressive vertical skin resection is particularly helpful in cases of pseudoptosis, where the lower pole of the breast is excessively prominent. As in any other breast reduction techniques, vertical scar mammaplasty works most easily in moderate-sized breasts with good tissues and elastic skin in young nonsmokers. A patient with normal and stable weight is preferable to an obese patient whose weight is constantly fluctuating. Juvenile patients are more prone unpredictable and often hypertrophic scar formation, and all efforts should be undertaken to keep scars as short as possible.

When is the Vertical Mammaplasty Unsuitable or Contraindicated?

Patients with large breasts, where the amount of tissue resection exceeds 1000 g per breast, and older patients, where skin has lost its elasticity and the breast has been replaced by adipose tissue, are not good candidates for this technique. In these cases, the amount of skin that has to be resected is too great, resulting in the classical inverted T-shaped scar. Another point of concern in those patients is the loose and flaccid tissue that can lead to early ptosis and lack of projection of the breast.

Patients with inelastic skin, even if the reduction is moderate, have a high risk of a residual excess of skin, and the patients have to be informed of the possibility of a small scar in the inframammary fold to obtain a nice redraping of the skin.

In the Hands of a Young Surgeon, Which Pattern Should be Used in Reduction Mammaplasty?

As far as the vertical scar in Lejour's technique (superior pedicle) is concerned, one must admit that some patients do not accept the aspect of the vertical scar with multiple wrinkles in the early postoperative period. Furthermore, scar correction at the bottom of the vertical scar is needed for many patients in our experience. The vertical technique is far more than just a scar; it is a concept. Breast shaping and modeling are the most important elements of this technique. We believe in scar reduction, but it should not be done at the cost of a high rate of wound dehiscence and scar revision. The vertical scar can be ended easily with a short horizontal scar if needed. However, in patients who have poor skin quality or long-lasting breast hypertrophy like elderly patients, a short inverted T scar will be more appropriate. Designing the inverted T at the end of the operation provides better scar placement with minimal extension of the scar to the sides. In addition, the skin excess at the inferior part of the breast can be excised in the form of an L or a J, in order to avoid any medial extension of the scar at the IMF.

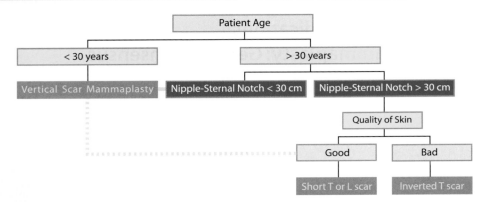

Fig. 15.1. Algorithm for planning scars in mammaplasty procedures

Moreover, respecting the IMF and using the superficial fascia as we described in Chap. 9 will help to obtain a better definition of the IMF.

My personal algorithm in scar selection is summarized in Fig. 15.1. I choose vertical scar mammaplasty in all patients under 30 years old. These patients usually have good skin quality, and skin retraction is expected. In very large breasts (more than 1000 g), secondary revision of the vertical scar is more likely to be necessary (see Chap. 14).

When the patient is over than 30 years old, I look first at the nipple-to-sternal notch (N-to-SN). If the N-to-SN is less than 30 cm, I choose a vertical scar technique. If this distance is more than 30 cm, I look at the quality of the skin and smoking history. If the skin is still elastic and there is no smoking history, I choose an L or J scar or short inverted T scar. However, a vertical scar can still be chosen if the surgeon has a large experience with the vertical scar technique. If the patient has nonelastic skin associated with strae marks and/or heavy smoking history, I choose an inverted T scar, which is designed at the end of the operation, in order to put the scar exactly in the new IMF.

By using this algorithm, any surgeon can achieve a good result with a minimal scar revision rate. It is extremely important to discuss these options with the patient during the preoperative consultation. The patient will be happier with the outcome and will more easily accept any necessary corrections later on.

Subject Index

R

Resection 18, 63
– „en bloc" 17
– horizontal 18
– keel 99
– vertical 18
– vertical wedge 20
– wise type 20
Retromammary space 77

S

Scars 126, 133
Septum, horizontal 2, 15, 76, 85
Seroma 44, 70, 126, 137
Skin
– brassiere 25
– closure 91
– excess 112, 134
Solutions 123
SPAIR (short scar periareolar
   inferior pedicle) 49

T

Tail of Spence 1
Taping 69
Thorek amputation 40
Two-finger maneuver 86

W

Wise pattern 25, 49